DEATH WITH DIGNITY

DEATH WITH DIGNITY

A New Law Permitting Physician Aid-in-Dying

Robert L. Risley

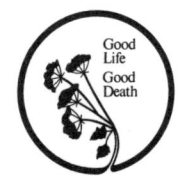

The Hemlock Society
P.O. Box 11830
Eugene, Oregon 97440

Death With Dignity © 1989 by Robert L. Risley.
All rights reserved. Printed in the United States of America.
No part of this book may be used or reproduced
in any manner whatsoever without written permission
except in the case of brief quotations embodied in
critical articles and reviews.
For information address
The Hemlock Society
PO Box 11830
Eugene, OR 97440.

Library of Congress Cataloging-in-Publication Data
Card number 89-061979

ISBN 0-9606030-8-5

KF
3827
.E87
R57
1989

Contents

CONTENTS ii

About the Author v

Introduction and Perspective vi

Acknowledgments xii

CHAPTER ONE.   THE NEED FOR CHANGE 1

   A Slight Legal Change Needed to Permit A Good Death 3

   The Recommended Change is Consistent
   With the Trends of Case Law 4

   Freedom of Choice Compels Legal Change 7

CHAPTER TWO.   EXISTING LAW IN THE UNITED STATES 11

   Case Law in America 11

   Living Will Statutes in America 31

   Durable Power of Attorney
   for Health Care Statutes in America 34

CHAPTER THREE.   LAW IN THE NETHERLANDS 37

CHAPTER FOUR.   THE DEATH WITH DIGNITY ACT:
                         HOW IT WORKS 47

   The Directive and the Conditions 48

   Protection of Physicians 49

   Reasonable Fees 49

Limitations 50

CHAPTER FIVE.   REPLIES TO OBJECTIONS 51

    Conceptual Objections 51

        1. The Law Would Be Abused 52

        2. Erroneous Diagnosis and Prognosis 55

        3. Right-to-Die Will Become a Duty to Die 56

        4. The Patient/Physician Relationship Will Be Weakened 57

        5. Physicians Should Not Be Executioners 59

        6. A New Law Is Unnecessary 60

        7. Euthanasia Is Being Abused in Holland 61

        8. Physicians Who Administer Aid-in-Dying
           under the Death with Dignity Act, if Enacted,
           Will Violate the Hippocratic Oath 61

        9. Legalizing Physician Aid-in-Dying Is
           the First Step on a Slippery Slope 63

      10. We May Become Nazi Germany if We Adopt
          The Death with Dignity Act 64

    Specific Objections to the Death with Dignity Act 65

        1. The Law Is Not Limited to Persons in Intractable Pain 65

        2. The Law Is Not Limited to Cases Where
           All Treatment Option Have Been Exhausted 66

        3. Physicians Cannot Determine Whether or Not
           Death Will Occur in Six Months 66

4. Surrogate Decision Making Is Inappropriate 67

  5. The DDA Does Not Go Far Enough Because
     It Does Not Apply to Quadriplegics or to Persons
     in a Persistive Vegetative State Who Are Not Terminal
     and Have Not Signed a DDA Directive 69

CHAPTER SIX. OUR ATTEMPT AT CHANGING THE LAW:
              THE TASK AHEAD. 71

  Prelude to Change: Options 71

  Efforts, Past and Present 74

  Our Task Ahead 79

APPENDIX A
The Death with Dignity Act 83

APPENDIX B
Summary of The Death with Dignity Act 101

About the Author

ROBERT RISLEY, an attorney, is the founding partner of a six-member Los Angeles law firm. Mr. Risley is also the author of the 1987 booklet, "Humane and Dignified Death—A New Law Permitting Physician Aid In Dying." Mr. Risley became involved in the right-to-die issue following his wife's death of cancer in the Bahamas in December 1984.

Along with colleagues, he drafted the Death with Dignity Act (formerly called the Humane and Dignified Death Act) and founded Americans Against Human Suffering, a national political action organization dedicated to enacting state laws which permit physician aid-in-dying for the terminally ill on request. Mr. Risley is a past president of Americans Against Human Suffering (AAHS) and is now chairman of its board of directors. The organization has 27,000 supporters throughout the United States, Canada, Australia, and Europe. Its offices are located in Washington, D.C. and Glendale, California. (P.O. Box 11001, Glendale, CA 91206.)

Introduction and Perspective

Those of us in society who want to change legal sanctions existing from time immemorial have a great challenge ahead. *"Thou shalt not kill"* is a basic edict of civilization. It is enshrined in the codes of every religious and legal system in both Eastern and Western societies. There is no more fundamental proposition.

However, the legal change that we seek, embodied in the Death with Dignity Act (DDA), is equally fundamental. It involves love and caring enough to permit dying people to end their suffering with the help of a physician rather than being forced to endure the agony of the dying process to the bitter end. It involves letting loved ones go when they are ready. It involves letting patients go when they are ready.

The challenge is worthy because everyone should be free to choose the time and place of his or her own death at life's end if they wish, and because everyone should have the fundamental right to control his or her own destiny.

The challenge to our American ancestors was equally imposing. In choosing to control their destiny they prevailed, as Americans are now free to worship, free to express their ideas, free to petition their government for redress of grievances, and free to send their children to schools of their own choice.

We take pride in these freedoms so hard to achieve. But the fight to achieve control over our own destinies at life's end is only now coming to the fore.

The right-to-die issue cuts across every discipline: philosophy, religion, morality, ethics, medicine, history, literature, the arts and the sciences. However, in order to be won, the issue must be recognized as essentially political; the struggle must be debated and resolved in the political arena through the democratic process. Success will require sacrifice of the time, talent and money of thousands of socially-conscious, concerned Americans.

Many battles long preceded the efforts of Americans Against Human Suffering, which was founded in 1986 to change state laws to permit physician aid-in-dying for the terminally ill. These were legal battles between traditional concepts of preservation of life and egalitarian concepts of personal autonomy and freedom of choice. Battles were waged in trial and appellate courts throughout the country and in state legislatures.

The court cases clearly established the right to bodily integrity, confirming that the basic right of self-determination includes the right to die, and that it overrides the state's duty to preserve life. Living will statutes have been enacted, giving individuals the right to instruct health-care professionals when life-support systems and extraordinary measures are not to be employed. Advocates of individual freedom of choice have, with few exceptions, won their battle to legalize "passive" euthanasia. But the battles for active euthanasia, if, indeed, the two can be logically separated, are only now developing.

The leading proponent of active voluntary euthanasia in North America has been the National Hemlock Society, which was founded in Los Angeles in 1980. For its first five years, the Society worked to raise public consciousness by publishing books and newsletters, by holding national and international conferences, and by giving frequent media briefings. The Hemlock Society has been and remains today the intellectual leader of the movement, emphasizing research about patients' rights and death and dying, publications on the subject, and public education.

The founder of Americans Against Human Suffering, Los Angeles attorney Robert Risley and his then law partner, Michael White, began drafting the DDA in early 1985. They soon learned of the Hemlock Society and contacted Derek Humphry and Law Professor Curt Garbesi. Thereafter joint efforts were made in advancing the concept in various forms.

As noted, the preceding legal battles and court cases all relate to what is commonly referred to as "passive" euthanasia, i.e., the right of an individual patient to order withholding or removal of life-support systems, thereby enabling the dying process to take its natural course. Americans Against Human Suffering's efforts to qualify the DDA by initiative petition in California for the November 1988 general election was the first time the concept of physician aid-in-dying for the terminally ill—"active euthanasia"—has been pursued, except in the Netherlands. Even there, the criminal code has not been changed. Instead, courts have carved out a judicial exception to prosecuting physicians for mercifully ending their patients' lives, but only when there is an enduring patient's decision and request, coupled with unbearable pain.

In America, the "initiative" process provides the only realistic vehicle for achieving the legal right of free choice at life's end, even though two-thirds of Americans favor physician aid-in-dying. This is because legislators avoid controversy where possible. They keep their jobs by accommodating the demands of vocal minorities and well-heeled special interest groups.

Several of these special interest groups are opposed to active euthanasia. Extraordinary efforts have already been made by AAHS to find legislative sponsors in several states. Only one California legislator agreed to sponsor comprehensive right-to-die legislation, including active euthanasia, but later backed out. While some may argue that it is preferable for the concept of active euthanasia to develop in the courts, building on a case-by-case basis, such a route would take many years and would initially be without safeguards, sanctions, and a developed method or procedure.

Moreover, in nearly every reported right-to-die appellate or state supreme court opinion already decided, appellate justices have urged legislative action. They rightfully point out that it is the duty of the legislature to develop specific policy and guidelines to minimize the risk of abuse. Unfortunately, their urging has fallen on deaf ears. As a result, AAHS, the Hemlock Society, and many individual lawyers, physicians and citizens throughout the country have responded to the need to act by developing a coalition of backers to pass the DDA by initiative in states where the process is available, and later in state legislatures where there is no initiative process.

Contrary to what some believe, the DDA honors the oft-quoted sanction "Thou shalt not kill," precisely because physician aid-in-dying for the terminally ill is not killing. To kill is to end the life of someone who wants to live and does not want to die.

For a terminally ill person who has requested help to end their suffering, the death knell has already been sounded. The killer is the disease or the trauma, not the physician. Here, the physician's help in dying is the highest, most compassionate kind of humanity. That is why physicians often help their patients die, but the help is provided surreptitiously because it is a crime. It shouldn't be a crime. The law must be changed.

In brief, this book describes the DDA and the 1988 attempt to qualify it by initiative in California. It describes the case law as it exists in the United States and in the Netherlands. It sets out objections to the Act leveled by critics and gives replies to these objections. It also describes the future plans of action.

In 1990 and 1991 the Hemlock Society of Oregon is actively campaigning to get the Oregon version of the Death With Dignity Act passed into law. The Hemlock Society of Washington State is developing an Initiative to the Legislature for 1991 to put the same law on the statute books. Attempts to make it law in California and Florida are slated for 1992.

Acknowledgments

Several friends have made enormous contributions in the writing of this book. Lloyd Egenes, a long-time friend and San Francisco lawyer, provided invaluable editorial criticism and suggestions. Alan Johnson, a retired professor living in Palm Springs, also provided editorial comment and invaluable suggestions, including extraordinary help in the preparation of Chapter Six.

I am especially thankful for the extraordinary editorial efforts of Ann Wickett, who shared her valuable time and talent to improve my work. I am also grateful to Professor William Sullivan of the USC Dental School, in his review of the manuscript and several invaluable suggestions.

Professor Marvin E. Newman of the Rollins School of Law in Florida was largely responsible for the contents of Chapter Three on Law in the Netherlands. Professor Newman took a sabbatical to the Netherlands where he witnessed and experienced legal active euthanasia firsthand. He studied the system, and interviewed treating physicians and patients.

I would also like to thank Jean Harmon, Grace Terauchi and Angela Guild for reading my illegible handwriting, and for listening to my garbled dictation.

I am grateful to my wife, Rosemary, for her patience and understanding while I was sequestered with journals, legal cases, statutes, and public survey polls.

Chapter One
The Need For Change

Science, medicine, and modern health care have nearly doubled life expectancy in the last fifty years. Cure, control, and prevention of disease have led the way. We are thankful for these marvelous advances, since many years of meaningful and productive life have been added for most people.

Yet along with increased longevity and the wonders of modern medicine, new problems have been created. The body can be kept "alive" long after the brain is dead. Or, a brain can still function in a terminally ill, pain-racked body, where agony is simply prolonged artificially by life-sustaining procedures.

Because the life expectancy of Americans and of most people in other Western countries has nearly doubled since the 1940's, the circumstances at death are dramatically different. Recent advances in science and medicine have resulted in new and increasingly complex realities facing nearly all of us when we die.

Today, 80% of Americans die in a hospital or other health-care facilities and under the control and management of a physician. Fifty years ago, only 20% of Americans died in a hospital or other health-care facility; most died at home. Extensive health care and treatment have become a new fact of American life at life's end.

Why has this happened? The answer is clear. We all want to be healthy. We all want the benefits of a physician's training and skills, we want a nurse's help and care, and we want the relief and healing that medication provides. We want all the healing arts so we may live as long as possible. Therefore, it is only natural that we seek out their services.

However, when we enter a hospital or other treatment facility, the medical system takes over, and in many cases we lose control of our lives. The strong and the knowledgeable take over, and patients are expected to defer to decision-making by the medical staff.

When we enter a hospital for the last time, we may have the strength, possibly the resources, and technically, the legal right to end our lives if we wish. But at that point our objective is to get treatment and cure.

However, physicians cannot always cure us, and as the dying process progresses and accelerates, we often lose the strength to help ourselves. Moreover, most people lack the knowledge and the means to end their own lives in a way that is acceptable to them. Nor do they possess the license needed to obtain life-ending substances, even if they knew how to use them. Therefore, they need help, but can't legally get it.

Thus, while science and medicine have changed the condition of our existence at life's end, the law has remained uncompromising. It prevents us from obtaining someone else's help, even that of a doctor who, at the patient's request, is willing to end a painful existence which has become intolerable.

The irony is that this is true despite the belief of over 80% of Americans that it is proper to remove machines used to keep terminally ill persons alive. The overriding majority of Americans now favor physician aid-in-dying. All recent polls consistently demonstrate this revised public attitude.

Such a change in attitude is reflected in the media as well as public polls. For example, the number of television dramatizations revolving around the right-to-die issue has risen dramatically in the last few years. In January 1987, Robert Young portrayed Roswell Gilbert, the engineer who shot his wife of 40 years, who suffered from Alzheimer's disease and osteoporosis, on NBC. This remarkable film was repeated on television in June 1989. ABC followed in April 1987 with "When the Time Comes," the story of a 30-year-old woman dying of cancer. She asked her childhood sweetheart to help her obtain life-ending drugs after her husband had categorically refused. Subsequently, in October on NBC, Raquel Welch played a victim of Lou Gehrig's Disease who wished to die on her own terms. As seen, the right-to-die issue flooded television, radio, newspapers, and magazines in 1987 and 1988. This is in stark contrast to the 1960's and early 1970's when the subject was literally taboo.

A Slight Legal Change Needed to Permit A Good Death

Reflecting the change in public attitudes toward the right to die, the proposed Death with Dignity Act (DDA) statute is really an extension of the laws existing in 38 American states and the District of Columbia where living will statutes exist. More importantly, the change that the DDA will bring simply legalizes what is *surreptitiously done* every day.

According to a survey of California physicians conducted by the Hemlock Society in 1988, 27% of doctors surveyed said they had helped patients die on request on more than one occasion. While it's gratifying that some doctors do help their patients die if asked rather than permit them to continue a painful existence, the help which doctors provide should be done openly, with safeguards, and clearly under the patient's control and direction. Helping a patient die should not be done surreptitiously.

As noted, 38 states and the District of Columbia have "Living Will" statutes which permit patients to end their lives by directing health-care providers to withhold or remove life-support systems. A living will is a document signed and witnessed well in advance of the onset of the dying process or end-stage disease. It is usually valid for seven years. These documents instruct health-care professionals about the appropriateness of extraordinary measures and life-support systems for the patient.

In some states, the living will can include instructions to

withhold systems which provide hydration and nutrition. If the patient is being nourished and hydrated through either an intravenous tube, nasogastric tube, G-tube or similar device, the patient will probably die of starvation or dehydration when these tubes are removed. If the patient is on a respirator, when it is removed, he or she will die by suffocation. These instructions which are permitted under present law in most states are not appealing. Indeed they are frightening. In many cases they doom the patient to a horrifying dying process.

Needless to say, the more humane way is to permit physicians to use analgesics, sedatives and anesthetics, allowing the patient to die in a dignifed and serene manner, as he or she has requested. When used in the proper dosage, these substances will completely and painlessly suppress respiration to bring a good life to an end with a good, peaceful death.

What makes a good death? This is a highly personal and individual matter. Consider the following: A good death is a painless and peaceful exit from life. If suffering and pain are present and the patient finds them intolerable, a good death involves self-deliverance with trained professional help.

A good death also involves the ability to choose, to control, and to be as autonomous as possible. A good death is one where there is time to discuss the decision with those we love, to be able to say a fond farewell, and to celebrate the closing of a worthwhile life with a gentle death at the time and place of our own choosing.

The Recommended Change Is Consistent with the Trends of Case Law

The right to withdraw artificial life-support systems from brain-dead patients has been increasingly tested in courts throughout the country and has been vigorously debated. In response to the growing number of cases, guidelines have been developed by state legislatures, the courts, and the medical profession to help determine exactly when it is appropriate to remove artificial life supports. It is more easily accomplished when a patient has signed a living will or a durable power of attorney for health care and has made known his or her wish before life-support systems are needed.

However, not until recently have guidelines been discussed for active euthanasia that would permit a competent, terminally ill adult to request and receive physician assistance-in-dying. Shouldn't a dying adult who is not on life-support systems be spared physical pain, mental anguish, indignity, loss of control, and the humiliation of withering away? Shouldn't such a competent person be entitled to active assistance in dying by the same medical professional who not only was unable to arrest or forestall the terminal illness any longer, but may unwittingly be prolonging the suffering?

It is fundamental under existing law that a thinking adult patient must give consent before medical treatment is rendered: that he or she may refuse treatment. The right to control the condition of one's life is a basic, private, and constitutionally-protected right.

Similarly, the right of a competent, terminally ill adult to select the time, place, and manner of his or her death is also a basic and private matter, and should be legally recognized. Mercy and human dignity demand that a terminally ill adult be permitted freedom of choice and, if he or she so elects, be permitted the aid of a physician to die a humane and dignified death.

Under living will statutes, and under court decisions throughout the country, patients have the legal right to end their lives by ordering withdrawal of life-support systems. Increasingly, patients' DNR (do not resuscitate) orders are being honored. Many people refer to this as "passive" assistance in dying. However, patients who are dying of relentless and painful illnesses, such as cancer or AIDS, and who are not on life-support systems, do not have the same legal right. They are not allowed to die by choice, because such assistance would require "active" aid-in-dying. Although as previously mentioned, doctors do occasionally (and surreptitiously) help patients die on request, nevertheless, nurses and physicians fear civil and criminal prosecution when they do help. They fear being charged with homicide or assisted suicide, as has happened in several instances.

Yet dying patients who are not on life-support systems should have the same right as the terminal person in the next bed who has requested that life-support systems be withheld. Cancer or AIDS victims may be subject to equal or even greater pain and indignity, but because they are not on life supports, are required under present law to suffer to the bitter end.

There is a better way. It is possible, through the proposed DDA, to accommodate a person's wish for aid-in-dying with proper ethical, medical, and legal safeguards. The Act has been carefully drawn to meet the needs of dying patients, their families, and the medical profession, as well as society as a whole.

This bold effort to change the law is consistent with the trend of legal changes as it moves against age-old sanctions and taboos. Not least important, there is a growing body of moral persuasion and legal opinion supporting this proposed new law. The concurring opinion written by Judge Lynn Compton in the case of *Bouvia v. Superior Court* (1986) 179 Cal.App.3d 1127, 1146-1148, is an example of this. Judge Compton concluded that:

> Fate has dealt this young woman a terrible hand. Can anyone blame her if she wants to fold her cards and say, I am out. Yet medical personnel who have had charge of her case have attempted to force Elizabeth to continue in the game. In their efforts they had been abetted by two different trial courts. . . .
>
> I have no doubt that Elizabeth Bouvia wants to die; and if she had the full use of even one hand, could probably find a way to end her life—in a word—commit suicide. In order to seek the assistance which she needs in ending her life by the only means she sees available—starvation—she has had to stultify her position

before this court by disavowing her desire to end her life in such a fashion and proclaiming that she will eat all that she can physically tolerate....

Elizabeth apparently has made a conscious and informed choice that she prefers death to continued existence in her helpless and, to her, intolerable condition. I believe she has an *absolute right to effectuate that decision*. This state and the medical profession, instead of frustrating her desire, should be attempting to relieve her suffering by permitting and in fact assisting her to die with ease and dignity. The fact that she is forced to suffer the ordeal of self-starvation to achieve her objective is in itself inhumane.

The right to die is an integral part of our right to control our own destinies so long as the rights of others are not affected. *The right* should, in my opinion, include *the ability to enlist assistance from others, including the medical profession in making death as painless and quick as possible*....

If there is a time when we ought to be able to get the government off our backs, it is when we face death—either by choice or otherwise. [Emphasis added.]

As so eloquently stated by Judge Compton, self-determination is the most basic of freedoms. Each of us has the absolute right to our own goals and values, as long as they do not infringe upon the rights of others. These rights include our right to die at life's end, and at the time and place of our own choice, whether by active or passive means. The law must so provide.

Freedom of Choice Compels Legal Change

Freedom to control our own destinies, and the freedom to choose the time and place of our own death is such a basic American concept that it is difficult to understand why this ideal is not enshrined in the constitution or laws of the land. Not so long ago, Americans fought and died for the freedom to worship as they wish, the right to send their children to schools of their choice, the right to be secure in their homes, and the right to due process of law. Now, Americans must fight to win the right to a humane and dignified death.

It is, simply, the right to be free to decide our own fate, a fundamental concept of Western civilization. As long as we do not infringe upon or endanger the rights of others, we should have the unfettered right to determine our own destiny, especially at life's end. Paternalistic concepts of what is right collectively must give way to free individual self-determination.

This freedom to choose is not suicide. It is not blind, irrational self-destruction. It is the rational ending of life where all hope is lost in the face of end-stage disease. Society rightfully works to prevent mindless and irrational suicide. None of us understands teen-age suicide, nor suicide at any age, when life is worth living for most of us. We know from personal experience that despondency and despair pass with time. State policy to prevent irrational suicide and preservation of life is valid and proper and should be fully advanced.

However, the ending of one's own life with the help of a physician when our life expectancy is only a matter of weeks is neither mindless nor irrational, but merely choosing between two kinds of death. It is choosing between the relentlessly painful dying process and release from suffering, a choice that the majority of people insists is one's final right.

Why, then, don't legislators change the law to permit physician-assistance in dying when most Americans support this right? Unfortunately, legislatures are oligarchies, responding primarily to the franchised and wealthy minorities in our society. Often they are not responsive to the majority's wishes. Attuned to negative criticism, they avoid criticism. This in turn means they shy away from controversial issues. No one will deny that voluntary euthanasia for the terminally ill is new, nor deny that it is controversial.

Certainly, there are risks associated with any legal change, and changing the law to permit physician aid-in-dying for those at life's end is no different than any other. Consequently, the DDA has been drafted with extraordinary care to provide all reasonable precaution to protect against the risks.

You will learn in Chapter Two that we have had the benefit of Living Will legislation and of court cases which have delineated issues and established requirements when life-support systems may be withheld or withdrawn. The justices writing the court opinions have frequently urged legislative action. Thus, it is now time to enact the DDA by initiative where possible, and to seek legislative sponsors in the two-thirds of the states which do not have an initiative process. Success will require a commitment of time, talent and money of thousands of socially-conscious, concerned Americans. Now is the time to join the effort.

Chapter Two
Existing Law in the United States

The right to die is based upon well-established legal and social principles. It is the basic right of every citizen to be free from interference. Our right to bodily integrity is carefully guarded by the law and cannot be violated unless we have given consent, or where there is evidence of criminal conduct. This right is fully developed in legions of court decisions, in state and federal constitutions, and in legislation.

Further, the majority of American states have now recognized that the basic right of self-determination and the right to bodily integrity include the right to die. This right is more important and outweighs the state's interest in the preservation of life, prevention of suicide, the integrity of the medical profession, and protection for innocent third parties. This chapter examines the major decisions which established the right to die and the structure and operation of living will and durable powers of attorney for health care statutes.

Case Law in America

The patient's right to refuse life-sustaining medical treatment has been upheld by virtually every state appellate court faced with the issue. Beginning with *In Re Quinlan* (1976) 70 N.J. 10, each of these states has followed an almost identical conceptual course of development in this area of the law. The case law has progressed in three stages. First, the cases established the patient's right to choose based on either the Constitutional right to privacy or the doctrine of informed consent, or both. Second was judicial recognition of the patient's or guardian's right to refuse life-support systems, usually a respirator.

Finally, the cases expanded the right to include removal of feeding tubes by the patient when competent, and by a surrogate when incompetent. The courts of the various states are basically in agreement in protecting individual patient autonomy and diverge only on the level of judicial or administrative intervention required for one to exercise the passive right-to-die.

The doctrine of informed consent is based on the right to be free from non-consensual physical invasions; this was recognized as early as 1891 in the United States Supreme Court case of *Union Pacific Railway Co. v. Botsford*, 141 U.S. 250. Here, the Supreme Court stated,

> No right is held more sacred, or is more carefully guarded, by the common law, than the right of every individual to the possession and control of his own person, free from all restraint or interference of others, unless by clear and unquestionable authority of law.

Recognizing that this right entitles us to refuse medical treatment, New York's highest court held, in *Schloendorff v. Society of New York Hospital* (1914) 211 N.Y. 125,

> Every human being of adult years and sound mind has a right to determine what shall be done with his own body; and a surgeon who performs an operation without his patient's consent commits an assault, for which he is liable in damages.

A modern statement of the law of informed consent can be found in the California case of *Cobbs v. Grant* (1972) 8 Cal. 3d 229. In that case, the plaintiff was admitted to the hospital for treatment of an ulcer and an operation was performed. Although the surgeon in the case explained the nature of the operation to the patient, he did not discuss any of the inherent risks. Complications later developed which necessitated two additional operations, the last being removal of half of the stomach.

The court held that a physician, in order to meet the standard of proper professional care, must divulge to his patient all information relevant to a meaningful decision-making process because "a person of adult years and sound mind has the right in the exercise of control over his own body, to determine whether or not to submit to lawful medical treatment." The court added that "unlimited discretion in a physician is irreconcilable with the basic right of the patient to make the ultimate informed decision regarding the course of treatment to which he knowledgeably consents to be subjected."

The *Quinlan* case is the most important right-to-die precedent in the United States, and was followed by every state court in which the issue arose. Moreover, the case led the way to enactment of "living will" statutes in many states.

Karen Quinlan was in a persistent vegetative condition, after having ingested alcohol and drugs on April 15, 1975, at the age of 21. She was on a respirator. A New Jersey trial court appointed Karen's father as her guardian. Subsequently, he requested that the court authorize the withdrawal of the respirator sustaining his daughter's life, a request opposed by Karen's doctors, the hospital, the County Prosecutor, the State of New Jersey, and Karen's guardian ad litem (a court-appointed guardian).

The trial court sided with Karen's doctors and refused the request of Karen's father. However, the New Jersey Supreme Court reversed the trial court, ruling that the constitutional right of privacy included the right to refuse treatment and that the decision could be made by a guardian.

As a result, Karen's respirator was removed. However, she did not die as expected and continued to breathe on her own. She was fed through tubes and given antibiotics to protect against infection, and she lived another ten years in this condition.

Of monumental importance, the *Quinlan* case established that the constitutional right of privacy, recognized in the

U.S. Supreme Court case of *Roe v. Wade* (1973) 410 U.S. 113, now encompassed the right of a patient to refuse medical treatment. After finding that Karen's right, as represented by her father, far outweighed the interests asserted by the state—namely preservation of human life and defense of the right of a physician to administer medical treatment according to his best judgment—the court determined that this right should not be discarded "solely on the basis that her condition prevents her conscious exercise of the choice." Although Quinlan had previously expressed distaste for heroic measures, the court gave her statements little weight as they were made while in good health. Instead, the court permitted Karen's guardian and family to render their best judgment as to whether the patient would exercise the right to refuse treatment in the particular circumstances.

However, the Court took extra precautions and required that the attending physicians determine that there was no reasonable possibility of the patient's ever emerging from the comatose conditon to a cognitive state. Finally, if the hospital Ethics Committee or similar body agreed with the prognosis, life-support systems could be withdrawn without any civil or criminal liability on the part of any participant.[1]

The following year, in *Superintendent of Belchertown State School v. Saikewicz* (1977) 373 Mass. 728, the Massachusetts Supreme Judicial Court held that a patient has the right to privacy "against unwanted infringements of bodily integrity in appropriate circumstances." Saikewicz was a severely retarded 67-year-old patient at a state mental health facility who had been diagnosed as suffering from acute myeloblastic monocytic leukemia, an invariably fatal disease.

The superintendent of the facility petitioned the probate court for the appointment of a guardian to make treatment decisions. The guardian and two physicians testified against administering chemotherapy treatment because the fear and pain Saikewicz would suffer outweighed the limited possibility of "some uncertain but limited extension of life." The

---

[1]These safeguards, among many others, are contained in the Death With Dignity Act.

probate court accepted the recommendation against treatment, and held that no treatment would be administered for the leukemia. Saikewicz died without pain nearly four months later from bronchial pneumonia, a complication of the leukemia.

The Supreme Judicial Court affirmed the lower Court's decision, stating:

> The Constitutional right to privacy... is an expression of the sanctity of individual free choice and self-determination as fundamental constituents of life. The value of life as so perceived is lessened not by a decision to refuse treatment, but by the failure to allow a competent human being the right of choice.

Next, the Massachusetts Supreme Court identified four important state interests against which the individual interest must be weighed: 1) preservation of life, 2) protection of innocent third parties, 3) prevention of suicide, and 4) promotion of the ethical integrity of the medical profession. The court found the first to be outweighed by the individual's interest in refusing unwanted bodily intrusions. It also held that the ethical integrity of the medical profession was not offended by withholding of treatment. The other two were inapplicable to this case.

The Massachusetts Supreme Court decision is remarkable because it rejected the approach of *Quinlan* which left the decision to the guardian, family, attending doctors, and hospital ethics committee. Instead, the Massachusetts Court ruled that future cases should be brought to the Probate Court for an adversarial hearing in which the Probate Judge has appointed a special guardian to represent the patient's interest and to present the judge with all reasonable arguments in favor of administering treatment to prolong life.[2]

Judicial intervention was later limited to Saikewicz's specific set of circumstances by the Massachusetts Court of

---

[2]The Death With Dignity Act follows the *Quinlan* lead to keep these personal decisions out of court.

Appeals in *In Re Dinnerstein* (1978) 6 Mass.App. 466. There, the court held that judicial proceedings were required only when the treatment offers a reasonable expectation of achieving a permanent or temporary cure of or relief from the illness, as compared to life-support mechanisms which only postpone death.

The first case permitting the removal of an artificial life-sustaining device from a competent, but terminally ill, adult, was *Satz v. Perlmutter*, decided in Florida in 1978.

Mr. Perlmutter was suffering from amyotrophic lateral sclerosis (Lou Gehrig's disease) and expected to die within two years when he sought removal of a respirator. The court considered the four state interests presented in *Saikewicz* and held that in the case of a competent patient all four were outweighed by the individual wishes of the patient.

Because all family members were in agreement, the Court found no injury to third parties. In rejecting the suicide concern, the court found that

> Mr. Perlmutter...really wants to live, but do so, God and mother nature willing, under his own power....Moreover, we find no requirement in the law that a competent, but otherwise mortally sick, patient undergo the surgery or treatment which constitutes the only hope for temporary prolongation of his life.

In ruling on the issue of medical ethics, the Court stated:

> It is all very convenient to insist on continuing Mr. Perlmutter's life so that there can be no question of foul play, no resulting civil liability and no possible trespass on medical ethics. However, it is quite another matter to do so at the patient's sole expense and against his competent will, thus inflicting never ending physical torture on his body until the inevitable, but artificially-suspended, moment of death. Such a course of conduct *invades the patient's constitutional right of privacy, removes his freedom of choice and invades his right to self-*

determine.[3] [Emphasis added].

The decision was affirmed by the Florida Supreme Court, which limited it to the facts presented.

The next major expansion of right-to-die law was initiated in the 1983 decision in *Barber v. Superior Court* (147 Cal.App.3d 1006), which established the right of a terminally ill patient to refuse nasogastric feeding and hydration.

As a result of withdrawing their patient's life supports, Dr. Barber and his colleague, Dr. Nejdl, were charged with murder and conspiracy to commit murder. Their patient, Clarence Herbert, had undergone surgery for closure of an ileostomy. Shortly after the successful completion of the surgery and while in the recovery room, Mr. Herbert suffered a cardiac-respiratory arrest. He was revived by a team of physicians and nurses and immediately placed on life-support systems. During the following three days, it was determined that Mr. Herbert was deeply comatose and not likely to recover. Tests revealed that Herbert had suffered severe brain damage, leaving him in a vegetative state.

Drs. Barber and Nejdl informed Mr. Herbert's family of their opinion that chances of his recovery were very slight. At that point, the family convened and drafted a written request to the hospital personnel, stating that they wanted "all machines taken off that are sustaining life."

As a result, the doctors ordered the respirator and other life-sustaining equipment removed. However, even after their withdrawal, Mr. Herbert continued to breathe without equipment while showing no signs of improvement. The family remained at his bedside and requested that Mr. Herbert not be disturbed, even objecting to certain routine procedures followed by hospital personnel in caring for comatose patients.

After two days, and after consulting with the family,

---

[3]It is this fundamental freedom of choice that is the basic reason to permit physician aid-in-dying for the terminally ill. Moreover, physician aid-in-dying is a more humane way to help end suffering than is removal of life-support systems to let people die of starvation, dehydration or suffocation. This passive method of dying is the only one permitted under case law and living will statutes.

Barber and Nejdl ordered removal of the intravenous tubes that provided hydration and nourishment to Mr. Herbert. From that point until his death, Mr. Herbert received nursing care which preserved his dignity and provided a clean and hygienic environment. However, someone complained to the authorities, and the Los Angeles District Attorney, thinking the doctors had killed Herbert, filed murder charges.

When the case was preliminarily reviewed in the municipal court, it was dismissed, only to be reversed by the superior court, which reinstated the murder charges. Drs. Barber and Nejdl appealed to the California Court of Appeals, which reversed again, and finally dismissed the charges.

The appeals court made clear that the responsibility for these decisions lies with the patient's family and doctor. The case emphasized that the wife was an appropriate surrogate decision maker. Like the court in *Quinlan*, the court concluded that a formal guardianship was not required. In addition, the court clearly stated that a physician is under no duty to continue treatment when there is no hope of a patient's recovery. Notably, the court held that nourishment by intravenous tubes was no different from a respirator or other artificial life-support equipment. This was the first time a court had ruled that nourishment and hydration were the equivalent of other life-support systems.

The trend was continued in the New Jersy case of *In re Conroy* (1985) 98 N.J. 321. Claire Conroy was an 84-year-old resident of a nursing home, afflicted with arteriosclerotic heart disease, hypertension, diabetes, and a gangrenous leg. Conroy's nephew and guardian petitioned a New Jersey Court for authority to remove a nasogastric tube. Although awake and conscious, Mrs. Conroy was unable to communicate and was expected to die within a year even if the nasogastric feeding were continued. If it were removed and the feeding stopped, she would die of dehydration in about a week.

As her guardian, Mrs. Conroy's nephew testified that his

aunt had always feared and avoided doctors and that he believed that she had never visited one until she became incompetent. It was for this reason that he refused to consent to the amputation of her gangrenous leg. The trial court permitted removal of the tube, reasoning that the focus of inquiry should be "whether life has become impossible and permanently burdensome to the patient. If so," the court held, "prolonging life becomes pointless and perhaps cruel."

The guardian ad litem[4] appealed, and while the appeal was pending, Conroy died with the nasogastric tube in place. The Appellate Court nevertheless reversed, holding that the right to terminate treatment was limited to patients who are brain-dead, irreversibly comatose or vegetative. The Court stated that withdrawal of nourishment from Mrs. Conroy would be "tantamount to killing her—not simply letting her die—and that such active euthanasia was ethically impermissible."

Conroy's nephew then appealed to the New Jersey Supreme Court, which held that life-sustaining treatment, including nasogastric feeding, may be withheld or withdrawn from elderly incompetent nursing home patients who are likely to die within approximately one year even with the treatment, if one of the following three tests are satisfied: 1) when it is clear that the particular patient would have refused the treatment under the circumstances involved (a subjective test); 2) when there is some indication of the patient's wishes, and when the burdens of continued life outweigh any benefits the patient can derive from that life (the limited objective test); and 3) when the pain and suffering associated with the treatment "clearly and markedly outweigh the benefits the patient derives from life" and "the patient is suffering from so much pain that prolonging his life would be inhumane" (the pure objective test).

In 1986, three more cases were decided which permitted the removal of feeding tubes, two from incompetent patients

---

[4]A guardian ad litem is a special guardian appointed by the court to represent the interests of an infant or an incompetent in litigation.

and one at the request of a competent, non-terminally ill patient. In *Corbett v. D'Alessandro* (1986) 487 So.2d 368, the Florida Appeals Court reversed the lower trial court, which had denied a request to discontinue nasogastric nutrition. Helen Corbett was in a persistent vegetative state, receiving nutritional sustenance solely through a nasogastric tube. Mrs. Corbett did not have a living will, nor had she designated, in writing, anyone to make treatment decisions for her. As so often occurs, Mrs. Corbett died prior to the trial judge's decision, still connected to the feeding tube.

The Appeals Court rejected the Trial Court's distinction between the withholding of food and water by the withdrawing of the nasogastric tube and the removal of "extraordinary life prolonging procedures." The Court stated:

> We are unable to distinguish on a legal, scientific, or moral basis between those artificial measures that sustain life—whether by means of "forced" sustenance or "forced" continuance of vital functions—of the vegetative, comatose patient who would soon expire without the use of those artificial means.

In *Brophy v. New England Sinai Hospital, Inc.* (1986) 398 Mass.417, the Massachusetts Supreme Court was asked to decide whether the substituted judgment of a person in a persistent vegetative state, and the artificial maintenance of his nutrition and hydration be discontinued, should be honored. The ward's wishes were supported by his wife who was also his guardian, and his family, but were opposed by his attending physicians and the hospital.

Brophy suffered a ruptured aneurism on March 22, 1983. Prior to that time, Brophy had been employed as a fireman and emergency medical technician. He enjoyed deer hunting, fishing, gardening, and performing household chores. After complaining of a severe, splitting headache, Brophy lost consciousness and was taken to the hospital. Surgery was performed a few days later to relieve an aneurism but was unsuccessful, and Brophy never regained consciousness, remaining in a persistent vegetative state. He was unable to chew or swallow and was maintained by a gastrostomy tube through which he received nutrition and hydration. According to a physician who testified at trial, the likelihood of Brophy's regaining cognitive functioning was substantially less than 1%.

In determining the Brophys' substituted judgment, the Court relied on several statements Brophy had made before the onset of his illness. Although he had never discussed specifically whether a feeding tube should be withdrawn in the event that he was diagnosed as being in a persistent vegetative state, Brophy had stated to his wife, discussing Karen Ann Quinlan, "I don't ever want to be on a life-support system. No way do I want to live like that; that is not living."

Brophy restated this preference after he had helped to rescue a man from a burning truck who died a few months later from extensive burns. Shortly after he said to his brother, "If I'm ever like that, just shoot me, pull the plug." Within 12 hours after being transported to the hospital following the rupture of the aneurism, Brophy stated to one of his daughters, "If I can't sit up to kiss one of my beautiful daughters, I may as well be six feet under."

The court agreed with earlier Massachusetts decisions, as well as those in other states in stating "The law protects a person's right to make his own decision to accept or reject treatment, whether that decision is wise or unwise." The court then balanced the state's interests against the right of the patient. In considering the state's interest in prolonging a patient's life, the court stated:

> We must recognize that the state's interest in life encompasses a broader interest than mere corporeal existence. In certain, thankfully rare, circumstances, the burden of maintaining the corporeal existence degrades the very humanity it was meant to serve.

The court held that Brophy's substituted judgment would be honored, and if the hospital refused, the guardian could transfer Brophy to the care of physicians who would comply.

The most significant decision since *Quinlan* was the 1986 case of *Bouvia v. Superior Court*, 179 Cal.App.3d 1172. The case was discussed briefly in Chapter 1. *Bouvia* was the first case in the United States to allow the withdrawal of a feeding tube from a patient who was neither incompetent nor terminally ill.

Elizabeth Bouvia was 28 years old when the case was decided. Since birth, she had been afflicted with severe cerebral palsy. She was functional for many years, but later became helpless. In 1986, she was a quadriplegic, and at 28 became a patient at a public hospital. Her physical handicaps had progressed to a point where she was completely bedridden. Except for mobility in a few fingers on one hand and slight head and facial movements, she was totally immobile, physically helpless, unable to care for herself, and was totally dependent upon others for all of her needs, including feeding, washing, cleaning, toileting, and turning. She could not stand or sit upright in bed or in a wheelchair, always remaining supine.

Besides cerebral palsy, she also suffered from degenerative and severely crippling arthritis that caused her continual pain. A tube was permanently attached to her chest that automatically injected her with periodic doses of morphine. The morphine relieved some but not all of her physical pain and discomfort.

She was intelligent and mentally competent. She had earned a college degree. She had married but the marriage was short-lived. She had previously suffered a miscarriage. She lived with her parents until her father told her they could no longer care for her, and then she stayed intermittently with friends and at public facilities. A search for a permanent place to live where she might receive the constant care she needed had been unsuccessful. She was without financial means to support herself and therefore was forced to accept public assistance for medical and other care. She expressed on several occasions the desire to die.

At the time of her hospitalization in 1986, Ms. Bouvia had to be spoon-fed. The medical staff concluded that she was undernourished because she had stopped eating due to nausea and vomiting. When her weight plummeted to 65 pounds, Ms. Bouvia's diet was changed from liquid foods given orally to tube-feeding imposed against her will and contrary to her written instructions.

The appeals court affirmed that everyone in California has the right to refuse medical treatment, which includes artificial feeding, and a right *not* to be kept alive at the insistence of others. Her care and treatment, even if considered wrong and fatal, were hers and hers alone. She knew the consequences of her request and decision and was willing to live with them. The forced insertion of tubes in her body against her wishes, the court held, "violated her constitutional rights."

As the court stated:

> Here, if force-fed, petitioner faces 15 to 20 years of a painful existence, endurable only by the constant administration of morphine. Her condition is irreversible. There is no cure for her palsy or arthritis. Petitioner would have to be fed, cleaned, turned, bedded, toileted by others for 15 to 20 years! Although alert, bright, sensitive, perhaps even brave and feisty, she must lie immobile, unable to exist except through physical acts of others. Her mind and spirit may be free to take great flights, but she herself is imprisoned and must lie physically helpless subject to the ignominy, embarrassment, humiliation and dehumanizing aspects created by her helplessness. We do not believe it is the policy of this state that all and every life must be preserved against the will of the sufferer. *It is incongruous, if not monstrous, for medical practitioners to assert their right to preserve a life that someone else must live, or, more accurately, endure, for "15 to 20 years."* [Emphasis added].

Each year, as more right-to-die cases are decided, the issue is no longer whether there is a right, but rather how it should be exercised. A trio of cases was decided by the New Jersey Supreme Court in 1987, two of them permitting the withdrawal of feeding tubes from incompetent patients and one allowing a competent patient to refuse the assistance of a respirator. The court relied on its decision in *Conroy* (discussed earlier), in permitting the withdrawal of feeding tubes, and delineated the procedures to be applied to patients who, unlike Clara Conroy, are neither terminally ill nor living in nursing homes.

In *Matter of Peter by Johanning* (1987) 108 N.J. 365, the patient was a 65-year-old nursing home resident in a persistent vegetative state, although not terminally ill. After having collapsed on her kitchen floor in October of 1984, Hilda Peter was resuscitated by paramedics but remained comatose in a persistent vegetative state. She began receiving nutrition and hydration from a nasogastric tube in January 1985.

Before the incident, Miss Peter had signed a power of attorney specifically authorizing her friend, Eberhard Johanning, to make all of her medical decisions. Hilda Peter had worked in a hospital for 10 years and had expressed to her friends her opinions about life-support systems. According to them, she had stated: "Under no circumstances would I want to be kept alive on a life-support system. I've seen too much of this at the hospital, and that's not for me." And, "When it's time to die and God wants to take me, I never want to linger around like my mother."

The court specifically rejected the argument that the withdrawal of artificial feeding directly causes death while the withdrawal of other forms of life-support only indirectly causes death, stating:

> Withdrawal of the nasogastric tube, like discontinuance of other kinds of artificial treatment, merely acquiesces in the natural cessation of a critical bodily function.

Thus, current law in New Jersey governing the withdrawal of life-sustaining treatment from a patient like Hilda Peter was set forth by the court. First, the surrogate decisionmaker should inform the state's office of the Ombudsman for the Institutionalized Elderly that a decision to forego treatment has been made. The ombudsman should then obtain two independent medical opinions to confirm the pathe patient's medical condition, the alternatives available, the risks involved, the likely outcome if medical treatment is discontinued, and assurance that there is no reasonable possibility of the patient's recovery to a cognitive, sapient state.

If there is clear and convincing evidence that a patient has designated a family member or close friend to make surrogate medical decisions, the ombudsman should defer any decision concerning life-support to the designated decision-maker. If no decision-maker has been designated, however, decisions may be made by a close family member. Only if there is no close family member available must a guardian be appointed.

The New Jersey court in *Matter of Farrell* (1987) 108 N.J. 335, stated procedures for the court when involved in withdrawing life-sustaining treatment from a patient living at home. Two non-attending physicians must examine the patient and make the same determinations that were specified in *Peter*.

Kathleen Farrell was another competent patient who asserted her right to die with dignity but for whom victory came too late. Stricken with Lou Gehrig's disease, Mrs. Farrell was admitted to a hospital where she underwent a tracheotomy and was connected to a respirator. She refused to allow the insertion of a nasogastric tube and the nurses were instructed not to resuscitate her. However, no issues arising from those directives went before the court. One year after first experiencing symptoms, Mrs. Farrell was released from the hospital because the staff could provide no further help for her condition.

After an experimental program that her husband characterized as "their last hope" had failed, Mrs. Farrell told him that she wanted to be disconnected from the respirator that sustained her breathing. Mrs. Farrell's doctor then arranged for a psychologist to interview Mrs. Farrell. The psychologist determined that Mrs. Farrell was not clinically depressed and needed no psychiatric treatment. She concluded that Mrs. Farrell's decision was informed, voluntary and competent.

On June 13, 1986, Mr. Farrell applied to the court for his appointment as special medical guardian for his wife with specific authority to disconnect her respirator. He also sought a declaratory judgment that he and anyone who assisted him in disconnecting her respirator would incur no civil or criminal liability. At the trial, one of Mrs. Farrell's physicians testified that she had told him, "I'm tired of suffering." After closing arguments, the trial court granted all the relief that Mr. Farrell had requested, but stayed its order pending appellate review.

On June 29, 1986, Mrs. Farrell died while still connected to the respirator. The guardian appointed for the Farrell children appealed to the New Jersey Supreme Court. The Supreme Court agreed to render a decision despite Mrs. Farrell's death, "because of the extreme importance of the issue, and the inevitability of cases like this one arising in the future," and affirmed the trial court's decision.

The New Jersey court in *In Re Jobes* (1987), 108 N.J. 394, required that the procedures stated in *Peter* (discussed on page 24) be followed before electing to remove a feeding tube from a non-terminal nursing home patient in a persistent vegetative state. Nancy Jobes was 25 and pregnant when she was in an automobile accident. During an operation to remove the fetus which was killed in the accident, she sustained an acute cardiopulmonary collapse. As a result, she suffered massive, irreversible brain damage and never regained consciousness. After five years, her husband and her parents requested that the nursing home in which she was a patient withdraw the jejunostomy tube which provided her with nutrition and hydration.

The court first attempted to establish Mrs. Jobes's medical preferences under the subjective test set forth in *Peter* and *Conroy*. The court stated, however,

> The probative value of prior statements offered to prove a patient's inclination for or against medical treatment depends on their specificity, their remoteness, consistency, and thoughtfulness, and the maturity of the person at the time of the statements.

Finding that "All of the statements about life support that were attributed to Mrs. Jobes were remote, general, spontaneous, and made in casual circumstances," the court ruled that the evidence was insufficient to meet the clear and convincing standard required by the subjective test.

In other words, because Mrs. Jobes had not made her preferences clear, the court deferred to the judgment of the family members and held that the court need not be consulted unless a health-care professional becomes uncertain about whether family members are properly protecting a patient's interest. The *Jobes* court followed the *Quinlan* lead of permitting the family rather than the court to make the decision, provided that health-care professionals did not object.

The most recent right-to-die decision was the case of *In Re Grant* (1988) 109 Wash. 2d 545, in which the Supreme Court of Washington issued an order permitting the withholding of life-sustaining procedures before the need for them actually arose.

At the time of the court's decision, Barbara Grant, age 22, suffered from the terminal illness known as Batten's Disease. This affliction, from which her two brothers also suffered, is a genetic, neurological, degenerative condition of the central nervous system. There is no known cure, and most victims die in their teens or early twenties. As the court described the disease's progression,

> ...victims...usually start life as normal appearing children. The first symptom is a problem with vision, followed by epileptic seizures and a loss of motor control which causes the child to stagger. Later, the child has speech difficulties. Eventually, the child can no longer walk or talk and is completely blind. Batten's disease also causes severe mental retardation, with intellectual functions progressively failing. The child develops difficulty with swallowing, caused by a loss of voluntary muscle control. Brain control of the heart and lungs deteriorates, initially causing irregular heart rate and breathing, and finally, cardiac or respiratory arrest. Ultimately, the child's vital functions fail, resulting in death.

Barbara Grant's condition followed the typical pattern of Batten's Disease. She was placed in a state school at age 14, and by age 21, she was confined to bed and had lost virtually all intellectual and cognitive functions. The school psychologist estimated her mental age to be between 2 weeks and one and a half months. By this time, the disease had also begun to affect the autonomic respiratory and cardiac regulation centers of the brain.

Barbara's mother, Judith Grant, sought an order from the Court authorizing the withholding of life-support systems; she opposed the state school's policy under which all measures necessary to sustain the life of an individual were used. If the necessary treatment was not available there, they then transported the individual to another hospital. Mrs. Grant testified that she believed her daughter would not want life-sustaining medical treatment because she had shown a dislike for taking medicine and having suction tubes used on her. The school chaplain also testified that in his earlier conversations with Barbara, she had expressed her understanding that she would die at an early age. It was his belief that Barbara had come to accept death and looked upon her life as a gift which she had a right to give back to God. As Mrs. Grant stated, "I think it's time for man to stand back and let God take over."

The trial court denied the motion, ruling it premature in that Barbara's condition had not yet degenerated to a comatose or vegetative state, and intrusive medical procedures were not yet necessary.

Yet the appellate court reversed the trial court, holding that in the absence of overriding state interests, a person has a right to have life-sustaining treatment withheld where he or she 1) is in an advanced state of a terminal and incurable illness, and 2) is suffering severe and permanent mental and physical deterioration. The court's order was as follows:

> The guardian, Judith Grant, natural mother of Barbara Grant, is authorized to approve and direct the *withholding* of life-sustaining procedures utilizing

mechanical or other artificial means including cardiopulmonary rescuscitation, defibrillation, the use of a respirator, intubation, the insertion of a nasogastric tube, and intravenous nutrition and hydration.

Further, the court held that prior judicial authorization is not required as long as the following criteria were met: 1) the patient is in an advanced stage of a terminal illness; 2) the patient would choose to refuse life-sustaining treatment, or the withholding of life-sustaining treatment would be in the best interests of the patient; and, 3) that members of the family, the physician, and the health care facility agree with the decision to withhold treatment.

Although the *Grant* decision was the first to permit a prospective order to withhold, it is significantly more restrictive than other states in that it limits the right to refuse life-sustaining procedures to terminally ill patients and requires the agreement of physicians and health care facilities.

The California Court of Appeal, in 1988, addressed the issue of whether a patient retains the right to refuse medical treatment after becoming incompetent in *Conservatorship of Drabick*, 200 Cal.App. 3d 185. On February 5, 1983, William J. Drabick sustained a severe head injury in an automobile accident. Drabick never regained consciousness and remained in a persistent vegetative state, receiving food and water through a nasogastric tube.

After Drabick had been comatose for nearly three years, his brother, who had been appointed conservator, petitioned the court for an order "authorizing the withholding of medical treatment, to wit, the permanent removal of nasogastric tubes, and the withholding of any other medical procedure or treatment utilized to deliver nutrition and hydration."

The court agreed with the majority of states in holding that judicial approval of a conservator's treatment decisions is not necessary unless the other interested persons disagree. When an interested person does seek the court's approval, the court limited its rules to determining whether the conservator has made a good faith decision based upon medical advice. The court approved the conservator's decision, stating

> William's severe head injury would have caused his death five years ago if his physicians had not replaced a vital function with a nasogastric tube. The decision to keep William alive immediately after his accident was the ordinary one that emergency care physicians make—to buy time in the hope that the patient can be cured. Now, however, after years of observation, William's physicians agree that he cannot be cured.

Although there was much evidence that Drabick would not have wanted to be sustained by a feeding tube, the court gave little weight to what it characterized as the patient's "prior informal statements." The court concluded that the conservator, acting in the conservatee's best interests, could consider the statements in good faith in making a decision in the patient's best interest.

Jeannine Gonzalez, who had lived with Drabick for the 12 years before his accident, testified to several conversations they had had about life-sustaining measures. Drabick stated emphatically that he would never want to be kept alive by a nasogastric tube as was his father, a victim of cancer of the liver. After being diagnosed as having polycystic renal disease, Drabick expressed his reluctance to use a kidney dialysis machine, stating "I won't be attached to a kidney machine. If I die, I die." According to Ms. Gonzalez, Drabick said, after seeing his father maintained by artificial life-support systems: "If anything ever happens to me, I would never want to be kept alive like that.... you've got to promise me that that's what would happen."

In short, appellate courts in New Jersey and Massachusetts, Florida and California, Washington, Arizona, and many other states, have now developed a judicial mandate, a body of law permitting Americans the right to die passively. This mandate is based on the constitutional right of privacy, the right of self-determination, the right to be free of bodily intrusion, and the right to be informed before consenting to any treatment.

This body of law conceptually supports active as well as passive euthanasia. Active euthanasia is, in many cases, far more humane. Many claim that removing life-sustaining systems that provide nutrition, hydration and oxygen, resulting in death by starvation, dehydration or suffocation, are not pleasant prospects. Moreover, many dying people are not on life supports, and they should be extended the same right to end their life peacefully and painlessly with the help of a physician. It is only proper, therefore, that these concepts be extended to active euthanasia.

Living Will Statutes in America

The first living will statute was enacted in California in 1976, just prior to the decision in the *Quinlan* case. California's Natural Death Act provides that any adult may execute a living will which is called a "directive." In a directive, one may state one's wishes that life-sustaining procedures be withheld or withdrawn in the event of a terminal condition.

In some states, "terminal condition" is limited to disease or illness. In others, like California, terminal condition also includes injuries. But the condition must be one which would result in death, whether life-sustaining procedures are used or not. Two physicians must certify that the patient is in a terminal condition, and the directive cannot take effect until 14 days after this diagnosis.

The directive must be signed by the declarant in the presence of two witnesses, and remains in effect for five years. However, if the declarant later becomes comatose or unable to communicate, the directive remains effective for the duration of the comatose condition or until the declarant is able to communicate.

Consistent with the majority of states, the California Act contains an exclusion for pregnant women. Specifically, if a patient who has signed a directive becomes pregnant, the document cannot be given effect during the course of pregnancy.

Like the living will laws in all other states, the Natural Death Act also provides that no civil or criminal liability will result from compliance by a physician or health facility with the requirements of the Act.

The major criticism of the Natural Death Act is that a doctor is not required to follow the directive unless the patient had already been diagnosed as terminally ill when he or she signed it. If the declarant was well when he or she signed it, it is considered advisory and need not be followed. It must be re-executed after learning of a terminal illness.

However, too often the patient becomes comatose or unable to communicate after signing the directive, and cannot restate his or her wishes. For example, a healthy person who makes his treatment preferences clear in a directive may be kept alive artificially against his will because he was rendered comatose by an unexpected car accident. Moreover, even those patients who are able to communicate are forced to endure an additional 14 days of unwanted treatment following the diagnosis of a terminal condition.

Another problem with the California law is that physicians are often reluctant to certify a patient as being in a terminal condition because they know that it will result in withdrawal of life-sustaining measures and eventual death of the patient. This is true despite the statute's civil and criminal immunity provisions. There is simply no guarantee that the patient's choice will be respected.[5]

As observed earlier, living will statutes are in effect in 39 states and the District of Columbia.[6] Most of these statutes are not nearly as restrictive as California's. For instance, they allow an individual to execute a binding directive prior

---

[5]The California legislature attempted to revise the California Natural Death Act in 1988, making the law more usable and bringing it into conformation with other states' statutes, but it was vetoed.

[6]The states which have enacted living will laws are: Alabama, Alaska, Arizona, Arkansas, California, Colorado, Connecticut, Delaware, Florida, Georgia, Hawaii, Idaho, Illinois, Indiana, Iowa, Kansas, Louisiana, Maine, Maryland, Mississippi, Missouri, Montana, Nevada, New Hampshire, New Mexico, North Carolina, Oklahoma, Oregon, South Carolina, Tennessee, Texas, Utah, Vermont, Virginia, Washington, West Virginia, Wisconsin and Wyoming.

to becoming terminally ill. The directive becomes operative once the patient is certified as terminally ill and is no longer able to make his decisions known.

About half of the living will laws contain the requirement that the patient be in a condition where death will occur shortly even if life-supporting treatments are employed. Thus, these states will not give effect to a living will unless the patient is so close to death that even artificial means will no longer keep him or her alive. The remaining statutes permit a living will to be followed so long as death is expected to result soon after life-sustaining measures are withdrawn. None of the living will statutes permits a non-terminally ill patient to decline treatment, even though the courts in many states have upheld this right. (See, for example, *Bouvia*, discussed on p. 22)

All of the statutes provide only that certain types of treatment may be withdrawn if already begun, or withheld if not yet begun. None of them permits the taking of active measures to end a patient's life. Normally the only mention of active euthanasia is a provision expressly prohibiting it. The majority of the statutes specifically exempt the withholding and withdrawal of nutrition and hydration, and some allow only mechanical and artificial treatment to be withdrawn or withheld.

Most living will statutes attempt to ensure the enforcement of the patient's wishes by requiring an uncooperative physician to transfer the patient to one who will comply with the directive. However, a few states treat the declarant's wishes as advisory. In those states, the doctor or health-care provider is not required to follow the patient's instructions.

Many statutes prevent the operation of a living will when a qualified woman patient is pregnant. Some of the states limit this exclusion to cases in which the fetus could develop to the point of live birth with the continued application of life-sustaining procedures to the mother.

Durable Power of Attorney for Health Care Statutes in America

The laws of eleven states[7] expressly authorize a Durable Power of Attorney for Health Care. Ten more states[8] have laws which imply that a Durable Power of Attorney for Health Care is permitted. These laws enable a person to give a power of attorney, which is valid for seven years, to a loved one or trusted friend, making that person an attorney-in-fact or agent. The purpose of these laws is to delegate decision-making authority for health care to another person so when the patient becomes incompetent or unable to express his or her wishes, the agent can do so.

The Durable Power of Attorney is binding, not simply advisory. It may be signed in advance of any terminal illness. Further, it allows the attorney-in-fact to refuse any treatment on behalf of the patient, rather than only life-sustaining measures such as the respirator. An individual may specify, within the power of attorney, his or her directions concerning specific types of treatment and services. The attorney-in-fact is required by law to act in accordance with this statement of desires. Most estate planners, lawyers and health-care professionals agree that the Durable Power is well conceived and effective. Durable powers legislation in other states is being considered.

The DDA combines the Living Will or Natural Death Act with the Durable Power of Attorney for Health Care's concepts, and permits an attorney-in-fact to be designated. The statutory form "directive" requires the individual patient to affirmatively make a very important choice about the authority of the attorney-in-fact. The attorney-in-fact can be empowered to request physician aid-in-dying, or the power can be withheld and exercised only by the patient in a face-to-face conversation with the treating physician. Decisions

---

[7]California, Colorado, Idaho, Illinois, Maine, Nevada, North Carolina, Oregon, Pennsylvania, Rhode Island, and Vermont.

[8]Arizona, Connecticut, Hawaii, Iowa, Maryland, New Jersey, New York, Texas, Virginia, and Washington.

made by the attorney-in-fact must be according to the directions or limitations stipulated by the declarant in the DDA directive. The declarant's wishes remain paramount.[9]

---

[9]If a patient is dying and in end-stage disease with a cancer that has metastasized, but the patient remains lucid and competent, which is often the case, then he or she can decide when the suffering will end, and can tell the doctor that the time has arrived for his final assistance. This is the way the new statute will work in every case where the patient is lucid and competent. However, if the patient was not lucid or was incompetent, an attorney-in-fact could make this final decision if and only if the patient had sufficient trust before becoming incompetent and specifically gave him or her that final authority.

Even after the surrogate decided that the time had come, the surrogate's decision would have to be reviewed by a three-person medical committee before the treating physician could follow the surrogate's instruction.

Chapter Three
Law in the Netherlands[10]

The Netherlands is the only country in the world where voluntary active euthanasia is openly permitted. The practice in the Netherlands began some time after 1973 when a physician was successfully defended against prosecution for aiding his patient to die on her request.

Since then, there have been over 300 cases reported to a public prosecutor's office. However, only seven or eight physicians have been prosecuted. Two of these physicians were convicted, and the others were acquitted. It is these cases that provide the body of law controlling the conduct of voluntary active euthanasia in Holland.[11]

The key to why this practice is accepted lies in the Dutch people's strong belief in self-determination—a belief so strong that it supersedes the influence of the church on this moral issue. Although the majority of the Dutch people profess faith in Protestantism or Catholicism, they are a more secular than religious people. The basic tenets of both the Protestant and Catholic churches clearly oppose any form of euthanasia, although recent polls show that two-thirds of

---

[10] Much of this chapter was excerpted with permission from a paper on VOLUNTARY ACTIVE EUTHANASIA, AN INDIVIDUAL'S RIGHT TO DETERMINE THE TIME AND MANNER OF DEATH by Marvin E. Newman, Americans Against Human Suffering Legal Advisory Board Member. Mr. Newman is a Professor of Law at Rollins College in Florida.

[11] Political concerns inhibit adopting a new euthanasia statute in Holland and these concerns are similar in the U.S. except for the initiative process in many states which gives expression to the popular will, even if legislatures, which are tradition-bound, will not.

Dutch society do not object to it.

However, this populist approval has not translated into legislative sanction. The majority Christian Democratic Party of the Netherlands, holding to its religious underpinning, opposes active voluntary euthanasia because it violates Scripture. The majority Liberal Democratic Party favors active voluntary euthanasia, but the position has given way to political realities.

In the 1987 election, the Liberal Democrats had to trade away their voluntary euthanasia stance in order to achieve other political goals. Because the mixture of religion and politics precludes the government of the Netherlands from taking any affirmative role in sanctioning voluntary euthanasia, the courts have been forced to set guidelines for justifying voluntary euthanasia. Arguably, Americans are more religious than the Dutch, but Americans, like the Dutch, also hold strongly to a belief in self-determination, the freedom of choice, and personal autonomy.

In 1973, the Criminal Court in the Netherlands, without suspending the criminal code, spelled out circumstances under which no sanctions would apply to a physician for assisting in voluntary active euthanasia. Although the Netherlands courts will convict physicians who assist their terminally ill patient in ending the suffering, the courts impose a more or less symbolic penalty.

Most cases, however, never reach the courts. Each year, approximately 5,000 people in the Netherlands decide to die with the aid of a physician, yet Dutch prosecutors pursue fewer than 5% of the cases that come before them. Those doctors who are prosecuted are often found guilty but not punished, on the theory that they took the only appropriate action under the circumstances. These cases are rarely appealed. However, two doctors were successfully prosecuted when culpability was established, according to Mr. Eugene Sutorius, a Dutch legal authority on euthanasia.

Emerging from the Netherlands courts' decisions on voluntary active euthanasia are guidelines under which physician aid-in-dying is acceptable. These guidelines apply to both the patient and the physician whose help is sought in ending the patient's life.

The first condition is that the patient's decision be voluntary. There must be clear and convincing evidence of enduring, free determination. Choosing in favor of euthanasia is voluntary only if made without coercion. The patient's motive for electing euthanasia is irrelevant, but factors such as pain, debilitation, emotional and financial burdens on loved ones, and the quality of remaining life may influence the decision. If possible, the request should be in writing as evidence that such a choice was a well-considered one.[12]

The second condition imposed by the Dutch is that the patient's decision be an informed one. In other words, the person involved must have adequate information as the basis for a sound understanding of the situation. Candid exchanges between doctor and patient ensure that the patient's decision is fully informed, as well as voluntary. Doctors carefully document all evidence of informed consent, often keeping a journal detailing all relevant facts.

The third condition is that the patient must face irreversible, protracted, and unbearable suffering. Notably, this guideline does not limit active voluntary euthanasia to the terminally ill. Thus, the Netherlands has accepted active euthanasia for chronically ill patients even though the illness is not terminal. Such a person may simply prefer not to live any longer. In one case, voluntary active euthanasia was approved for a patient who had attempted suicide thirteen times.[13]

The final condition is that there must be, from the patient's point of view, an absence of reasonable alternatives to alleviate the suffering. Most people choose among alternative courses on the basis of such factors as how many days

---

[12]A written and witnessed request is a prime requirement of the proposed Death with Dignity Act in America.

[13]In comparison, the Death with Dignity Act requires that the patient's decision be voluntary and informed, that the condition be incurable and irreversible, and it is limited to the terminally ill.

or months the treatment might add to their lives, and the nature and quality of that extended life. For example, someone might consider whether treatment would allow or interfere with pursuit of important goals, such as completing projects and taking leave of loved ones. Also relevant to the patient are the degree of suffering involved, and the costs—financial or otherwise—to the patient and others. The relative weight afforded each factor is ultimately the choice of the competent patient.[14]

Dutch case law has also generated conditions governing the assistance of a second party in accomplishing voluntary euthanasia. First, the assistance must come from a qualified physician. Second, the physician must act only after consulting another physician or expert who also approves the assistance. This approval must be independent and the result of the other party's own judgment. Third, the physician must exercise due care in performing the euthanasia. Finally, the euthanasia must be necessary or desirable from a medical point of view.[15]

To secure compliance with these standards, the Netherlands Public Prosecutor's office and quality-control medical inspectors have entered into an agreement regarding the handling of voluntary euthanasia cases. Although physicians are required to be frank in reporting the cause of death, euthanasia is nearly always reported as death by natural causes, to avoid any risk of prosecution as well as problems for the patient's family. The prosecution policy evidences the belief that decisions to prosecute for participating in voluntary active euthanasia should not run counter to the conditions for impunity developed in the administration of justice by the Netherlands courts.

---

[14]Alternative factors such as cost are not spelled out in the Humane and Dignified Death Act. These factors are left to the patient's discretion, provided that two physicians have confirmed the terminal condition.

[15]The Death with Dignity Act proposed for American states is in accord on the first three conditions. It does not encompass the concept of "medically desirable," as that condition imposes an outside third party's value judgment, and is unnecessary where the patient is terminal and treatment options are exhausted.

From 1982 through 1984, for example, 36 cases of euthanasia were brought to the attention of the Public Prosecutor. Of these cases, 78% were dropped. This illustrates the deferential approach to euthanasia cases that eventually led the Netherlands High Court to accept the *responsible* practice of voluntary active euthanasia. The Supreme Court decision, handed down in November 1984, is a good source for examining the legal theories behind sanctioning voluntary active euthanasia. It also illustrates the tough moral and ethical questions facing the doctor, the patient, and the patient's family.

Although only the physician who assists in euthanasia may face prosecution, the patient is the central figure in right-to-die cases. The patient's life, illness, suffering, wish to die, and death create every euthanasia issue. In the landmark case before the Netherlands High Court, for example, a 94-year-old woman who had always been a vital, mentally strong person, setting great store by her independence, had asked her doctor to help her die. At the time of the request, the woman lived in a home for the elderly. Her body functioned poorly and she could not walk or sit up. Speech was almost impossible, and she was totally dependent on the nursing staff for the most elementary activities. However, in this case, dependence did not preclude competence. The patient was fully conscious and deeply aware of her progressive degradation. Her understanding of her condition became acute as her failing health robbed her of her ability to communicate with those around her.

In the last week of this woman's life, her physical condition deteriorated sharply, leaving her unable to drink or speak. She lost consciousness for some time. After a slight remission, however, she urgently repeated to her doctor her previous requests for help in ending her unacceptable life. After long and exhaustive discussions between them, the physicians decided to administer a series of injections that would lead to the woman's death.

The first put her to sleep. The second, administered ten minutes later, sent her into a coma. A few minutes later, a final injection induced respiratory arrest and the woman was dead. The doctor then informed the police and the medical examiner about the euthanasia. Because the doctor refused to report the death as resulting from natural causes, criminal charges were brought. The judicial process that followed sheds light on the conflicts inherent in the application of voluntary active euthanasia.

The lower court dismissed the charges against the physician not only because it could not find the doctor's conduct undesirable, but because the doctor had also satisfied the highest standards of conscientiousness. Still, the Prosecutor's office appealed the lower court's decision. The Amsterdam Court of Appeal reversed, finding the doctor guilty.

The appellate court reasoned that it could not accept public opinion as sanctioning euthanasia in direct opposition to the Netherlands Criminal Code. Section 293 of the Code makes it a crime to deliberately take the life of another. The court rejected the physician's defense that under the emergency conditions his loyalty to his patient superseded his loyalty to the law.

In turn, the Netherlands High Court disagreed and quashed the appellate ruling. The High Court held that the appellate court should have carefully weighed the conflicting duties and interests of the physician and then made an objective decision as to whether or not his conduct was justified.

Therefore, holding that an emergency situation could have existed, the Court overturned the decision. Although the Netherlands High Court was under no obligation to state the reasons for its holding, it expressly stated that voluntary euthanasia cases should primarily be judged by legal, not medical standards. This choice indicates an intent to take the problem out of the courts and place it back in the discipline from which it arose.

Because the High Court of the Netherlands must refrain from inquiry into the facts and merits of cases, it is strictly limited to judging whether lower courts remain within the law and follow proper procedures. If a case is remanded, another Court of Appeal addresses the points of inquiry. The public prosecutor stopped pursuing the case against the physician before it went to the second appellate court.

According to the Court, voluntary euthanasia must be medically justified and judged under medical ethics. In determining justiciability, three questions must be considered. First, was the continued faltering health of the patient, disintegration of personality, and further deterioration and unbearable suffering to be expected? Because a personality factor is included, both physical and nonphysical suffering are relevant. There is no absolute requirement that the patient be terminally ill.

The second question is, could it reasonably be foreseen that a dignified death would no longer be possible? This question indicates respect for the conscious, dying human being as well as the living. Finally, were there any alternative ways, acceptable to the patient, to alleviate the suffering?

Although the answers to these questions must be based primarily on objective medical views, this is only the first judgment. The final determination as to permissibility remains a legal one and must, therefore, rest with society and the courts. If any reasonable doubt exists the Criminal Court may decide whether a physician's loyalty to the patient superseded loyalty to the law, so as to justify the physician's decision to assist in the patient's wish to die. The Netherlands High Court's decision may be justified by medical, ethical and legal standards without requiring amendment to the Netherlands Criminal Code.

For instance, after the High Court's decision, two district courts acquitted physicians who conformed with the High Court's standards. In another case, however, a district court convicted a physician who assisted in voluntary euthanasia and sentenced him to one year in prison. The court found the doctor, although well-intentioned, had been careless and negligent. In such a controversial issue as voluntary euthanasia, strict adherence to the guidelines is essential in the Netherlands as it is under the proposed Humane and Dignified Death Act.

While the Netherlands High Court was still considering the 1984 decision discussed earlier, the Dutch Medical Society set forth its own standards, similar to those generated by lower court decisions, for practicing voluntary active euthanasia. The report states that only a physician may act to terminate a life, but should never be compelled to do so. When a patient and doctor disagree about the propriety of euthanasia, the physician must allow the patient to contact another physician as soon as possible.

The Medical Society report also requires a physician to exercise due care in ensuring that the patient's decision is a voluntary, informed one that reflects a desire to end unbearable suffering. The report, however, does not fully explore the doctor's role in the patient's initial decision to choose death.

A patient can request aid-in-dying in one of three ways: First, a living will can indicate a person's refusal of life-support machines in order to achieve a dignified death. This is voluntary passive euthanasia. Second, a patient can request aid-in-dying during the course of an illness. Finally, the patient can reply affirmatively if the physician suggests that euthanasia might be appropriate in view of the patient's condition. Although many patients accept such a suggestion as a valid alternative, most physicians hesitate to initiate the suggestion. Some find it contrary to their personal views; others see it as a violation of their medical ethics.

Traditionally, a physician's primary duty is to preserve life and relieve pain. Arguably, then, suggestions of aiding those who wish to die is contrary to the Hippocratic Oath. Some medical philosophers read Hippocrates' writings as prohibiting a physician from ever helping a patient to die. Others note that Hippocrates held the patient's interests to be of supreme importance.[16] They view voluntary active euthanasia to end unbearable suffering as an act in the

---

[16]The entire oath is set out on pages 61-2 and is further discussed in the pages that follow.

patient's best interests. Consequently, they conclude that a physician who can do no more for a patient has an ethical responsibility to a patient's request to ease his or her passing.

The patient's family also plays an important role in the aid-in-dying decision. In fact, relatives of someone who chooses death may have the most difficult role. Some patients, especially older ones, hesitate to discuss euthanasia with their physician but feel more at ease discussing the subject with relatives.

If the request for help in dying comes solely from the family, however, it can often lead to the assumption that they, and not the patient, are actually behind the decision. In such instances, medical teams properly hesitate to carry out the euthanasia because reasonable doubt exists as to voluntariness.

Although the coalition government of the Netherlands, consisting of Christian Democrats and conservatives, does not support legislation to reduce the tension between the present criminal code and the developing practice of voluntary euthanasia, one small, liberal political party has introduced a bill to amend the present law. Under the proposed law, voluntary active euthanasia would no longer be an offense if it were practiced with due care for the benefit of a patient who is suffering unbearably or is terminally ill.

The proposed legislation incorporates most of the same guidelines set forth by the Netherlands, judiciary, the Dutch Medical Society, and the Government Commission on Euthanasia. Although the bill garnered popular support, populism typically plays second fiddle to the political realities in the Netherlands,[17] and no new legislation should be expected in the near future.

---

[17] The explanation of resistance to legislative change in American set out in Chapter Six is equally applicable to the difficulties in the Netherlands.

Chapter Four
The Death with Dignity Act: How It Works

As discussed in Chapter Two, the proposed Death with Dignity Act (DDA) was developed by combining and enlarging the California Natural Death Act (Health and Safety Code Section 7185-7189.5) and the Durable Power of Attorney for Health Care Decisions Act (California Civil Code Section 2500-2513). Under these statutes, adults can declare that they do not wish to be kept alive artificially by life-support systems and they can provide for the advance appointment of an attorney-in-fact or surrogate decision-maker to make health-care decisions, including withholding or withdrawing life supports, if the patient becomes incompetent.

The DDA would confer on all competent terminally ill adults the right to request and to receive a physician's aid-in-dying, when terminally ill, under carefully defined circumstances. In addition to combining the two existing California laws, the DDA also immunizes physicians and health-care workers from liability for responding to a patient's request for aid-in-dying, provided the request is written and conforms to the strict rules of the DDA. It also permits private hospitals to adopt policies precluding physician aid-in-dying in their facility.

The DDA provides that a competent adult patient may, personally or through an agent, request either (or both) passive and active voluntary euthanasia, provided the requirements of the DDA are met.

The Directive and the Conditions

First, a competent adult must sign an DDA directive in the presence of two disinterested witnesses. Witnesses *cannot* be beneficiaries, heirs, or creditors of the patient, nor can they be health-care providers. The witnesses must declare that the patient is competent. In this document, patients must specify that their lives not be prolonged artificially and/or that their lives be ended with the help of a physician upon request. They must also designate an agent to make health-care decisions in case they become incompetent. The agent is then permitted to request physician aid-in-dying, if specifically so empowered. The competent adult person may specifically deny the agent this power of decision in the directive by initialling a box.[18]

Second, patients must inform their families and indicate that they have considered their opinions. However, they still retain the right of final decision as long as they are competent. The directive is effective for seven years. However, the period is extended if the seven-year period ends while the patient is incompetent.

Several conditions must be met before a physician may legally comply with a patient's directive.

- First, the DDA directive must have been properly signed by a competent adult and properly witnessed.
- Second, it must not have been revoked. The directive can be revoked by being cancelled, defaced, obliterated, burned, torn, or destroyed by the signer or another person acting on the signer's direction. It can also be revoked by written revocation of the signer, expressly indicating his or

---

[18]See Footnote number 9, Chapter Two, which is set out here for convenience.

If a patient is dying and is in end-stage disease with a cancer that has metastasized but the patient remains lucid and competent, which is often the case, then he or she can decide when the suffering will end and tell the doctor the time has arrived for his or her final assistance. This is the way the new statute will work in every case where the patient is lucid and competent. However, if the patient is not lucid or is incompetent, an attorney-in-fact can make this final decision if and only if the patient had sufficient trust and specifically gave him or her that final authority.

Even after the surrogate decided that the time had come, the surrogate's decision must be reviewed by a three-person medical committee before the treating physician could follow the surrogate's instructions.

her intent to revoke the directive, signed and dated. The directive can also be revoked by verbal expression of the signer's intent to revoke the directive; revocation becomes effective only upon communication of that decision to the attending physician by the signer or by a person acting on behalf of the signer.
- Third, the action to be taken must fall within the seven-year, or longer, period allowed, as noted previously.
- Fourth, two licensed physicians must certify to a reasonable medical certainty that the patient is terminal, that is, death is likely to occur within six months.
- Fifth, one of the certifying physicians must be the treating physician, but the two certifying physicians must be independent of each other. That is, they may not be partners and workers in the same medical practice.
- Sixth, if the patient becomes incompetent after that certification, and if the final decision is made by the agent, the decision must be reviewed by a three-person ethics committee.
- Seventh, the treating physician, with the patient's consent, may order a psychiatric or psychological consultation if he or she is uncertain about the patient's competence to make the request for physician aid-in-dying.

Protection of Physicians

The initiative protects physicians, and other health-care workers acting under a physician's and hospital's instructions, from civil, criminal, and administrative (i.e., licensing) liability when complying with the patient's request(s) in the directive according to law.

Reasonable Fees

The DDA requires hospitals and other health-care providers to keep records and to report certain information to the Department of Health Services, but only after the death of the patient, and then anonymously. It also requires that physicians' fees for professional services be reasonable when the physician complies with the patient's directives.

Limitations

The DDA specifically forbids aid-in-dying to any patient solely because he or she is a burden to any other person, or because the patient is incompetent or terminal without having made an informed and proper DDA directive according to law.

The DDA does not change the law that makes aiding, abetting, advising, or counseling suicide a crime. It does not permit aid-in-dying to be performed by loved ones, friends, or strangers. It does not apply to children. Indeed, it does not affect anyone who has not voluntarily and intentionally completed and signed a properly witnessed directive according to law.

In summary, the proposed statute stipulates that an adult has the right to request and receive a physician's aid-in-dying under carefully defined circumstances. It combines the Natural Death Act and adds a Durable Power of Attorney for Health Care. It gives the adult patient the option of empowering or not empowering the attorney-in-fact to request physician aid-in-dying. It immunizes physicians, health-care workers, and hospitals from liability in carrying out a patient's wishes. In order to take advantage of the law, a competent adult person must sign the DDA directive. The full text of the Act is set out in Appendix A.

Chapter Five
Replies to Objections

Americans Against Human Suffering endeavored to qualify the Humane and Dignified Death Act (now called the Death With Dignity Act) by initiative in California for the November 1988 general election. During the effort, several objections were encountered. These objections fall into two categories. First were objections to the basic concept of physician aid-in-dying and voluntary active euthanasia, and second were technical objections to the DDA as written.

Conceptual Objections
Opponents of the DDA gave the following criticisms in voicing their objections: 1) the law will be abused, 2) physicians may be wrong in their diagnosis and prognosis, 3) the right to die may become the duty to die, 4) physician aid-in-dying will weaken the patient/physician relationship, 5) physicians should not be executioners, 6) a new law is unnecessary, 7) euthanasia is being abused in Holland, 8) a physician aid-in-dying policy violates the Hippocratic Oath, 9) legalizing physician aid-in-dying is the first step on a slippery slope, and 10) we may become like Nazi Germany if we adopt the DDA.

Each of these objections is explained, and a full response is given in the order listed.

1. **The Law Would Be Abused:**
   a. The principal objection to a law permitting physician aid-in-dying is that it may be abused: A patient's life may be ended for malicious, not merciful, reasons without his or her request or consent.

   This is a valid concern to all of us. Potential abuse of a law is always present, and the DDA is no different from any other law. However, law enforcement and the criminal justice system exist to identify, apprehend, and punish lawbreakers. We must rely in part on the criminal justice system to deter wrongdoing, just as we do to prevent homicide generally.

   However, the DDA has built-in protection from abuse. The principal protection in the DDA is that only licensed physicians are permitted to give aid-in-dying to the terminally ill patient who requests it. Widespread merciful euthanasia performed by friends or loved ones will remain illegal.

   The weak and the elderly who are most vulnerable to abuse are protected because licensed physicians are not likely for several reasons to abuse the law. Physicians are supervised by state licensing authorities, who in turn are responsible and authorized to discipline physicians.

   Such discipline and possible loss of their license is of significant concern to them. Physicians practice under a well-recognized code of ethics. They are partially controlled by peer pressure and review by colleagues, hospital staff and administrative guidelines. They are concerned about their reputation and controlled by their own conscience, not to mention the law.

   Moreover, a physician's economic interests generally run counter to a patient's request for aid-in-dying. It is axiomatic that since most physicians get paid for treating patients, the longer the patient lives, the longer the physician will get paid. If avariciousness is involved, the physician will keep the patient alive as long as possible to continue receiving fees and will not be motivated by economic reasons to end his or her patient's life.

   Ordinarily, the physician will comply with a patient's

directive to withhold or withdraw life-support measures or to give aid-in-dying out of compassion for the patient, as many physicians do today quietly and illegally at great risk to themselves. Under the DDA, the physician may lawfully assist a dying patient who requests help using the training, skill, and license which laymen do not possess. In complying with the patient's request out of compassion, the physician must conform strictly to the terms of the proposed act.

Strange as it may sound, permitting physicians to actively help their terminally-ill patients die, that is, to administer euthanasia, is safer and less likely to be abused than the present system of removing or withholding life-support systems and letting patients die, which is passive euthanasia. The reason that active euthanasia is less likely to be abused than passive euthanasia is that helping someone die is a direct and open deed. The morality and responsibility for the act must be faced squarely. The doctor will say to him or herself, "I am going to end this life as I have been requested. It is my responsibility."

Indifference in the face of this realization is nearly inconceivable. The experience of physicians in the Netherlands who have affirmatively helped patients die on request is that it is always a very emotional act.

The reverse is true of passive euthanasia, however, where a number of rationalizations or justifications can be used to excuse the physician of responsibility for ending the patient's life and to make the act less emotional. When life-support systems are removed, physicians can claim that they are "simply letting nature take its course," or that the patient is "now in God's hands and not my responsibility."

There is nothing wrong with this attitude and justification, as dying is nearly always beyond anyone's control. The physician who is legally permitted to affirmatively help a terminally ill patient die and decides to do so knows the consequences as well as the time, place and cause. He or she is not pulling a plug and then walking from the room and handing responsibility to nature or God. Rather, that physician is deciding to help a fellow human being ease out of this life knowing full well the measure of patient and doctor responsibility.

b. Some opponents say that irresponsible physicians may themselves abuse the law by sweeping away their mistakes and disposing of incriminating evidence if physician aid-in-dying is legally permitted for the terminally ill.

Our response is simple. Regrettably, mistakes are made today by doctors as well as the rest of us. We see evidence of this in the numerous medical malpractice claims and awards in courts throughout the country.

However, there is no evidence of physician abuse of living will statutes where physicians routinely remove life-support systems upon request, thus allowing the patient to die. Neither is abuse likely after the DDA is adopted because the numerous constraints mentioned above will prevail. Physicians now have the opportunity to conceal their mistakes under present law. If there is misconduct, it must be prosecuted by the appropriate authorities.

The celebrated *Barber* case in California, which resulted in the appellate court exonerating two doctors charged with murder, did not really involve abuse; the physicians were simply following the patient's and family's request to remove life-support systems. Drs. Nejdl and Barber's conduct was clearly correct because Clarence Herbert was dying and had the legal right to control his own destiny and his own body. They were not ending his life against his wishes. Had Dr. Barber accelerated Herbert's dying in the face of an express or implied wish to be kept alive, they would have been guilty of murder. Such was not the case.

If a doctor ends a life on his own initiative or discretion and without being requested by the patient to do so, he has committed murder. Although physicians can and do kill patients on occasion, they are invariably motivated by the human frailties of avarice, passion, mental derangement, or gross incompetence.

But most physicians simply do not murder their patients. Permitting them to help a dying patient to a peaceful death will in no way increase the risk of homicide.

c. Some opponents claim that affirmatively ending life is an abuse of nature.

If active euthanasia is an abuse of nature because it consists of our determining the time death will occur, as critics claim, then we are also abusing nature in a similar way when we engage in passive euthanasia. In both cases, we choose an earlier death in preference to a longer life—in one case by administering a lethal substance, in the other by discontinuing life-sustaining treatment.

Why is it an abuse of nature to determine the time of our own death when nature has given us autonomy, that is, the ability to choose? Is it not precisely this ability that gives special value and dignity to human beings? Is that not equally a part of human nature?

Autonomy, the freedom to choose, is a fundamental human value unique to human beings. It is the disease killing the patient, and many argue that artificial life supports are in fact the real abuse in not letting nature take its inevitable course. In avoiding that fate, we are electing to die in a manner befitting our dignity.

2. Erroneous Diagnosis and Prognosis:

Opponents of the DDA point out that physicians are fallible human beings like the rest of us, and may be mistaken in their diagnosis or prognosis of death. They say that sometimes doctors tell patients they have only a few months to live, but in fact some patients continue to live for years.

The DDA contemplates this criticism and requires a "second opinion." It specifically requires, as noted, that two licensed physicians agree that the patient is terminal.

However, even then, the statute recognizes that two physicians may be mistaken as well, and the patient must take this into account and be responsible for this possibility. The directive specifically provides:

> I recognize that a physician's judgment is not always certain, and that medical science continues to make progress in extending life, but in spite of these facts, I

nevertheless wish aid-in-dying rather than letting my terminal condition take its natural course.

In practice, physicians know "end-stage disease" when it exists. They know, for instance, that when a cancer is coursing through the body with massive metastatic process at work, death is only a matter of hours, days, or weeks. Physicians also know when treatment options have been exhausted. They should (and most do) inform their patients and families when this occurs. If there is any question about their opinion they inform their patient accordingly.

Moreover, they should inform their patients of any new "medical breakthrough" which may yet save their life. Armed with this information, the patient can make his or her own decision about continuing to endure the pain or indignities, or to request assistance-in-dying at the time, place, and manner of his or her own choosing.

3. **Right-To-Die Will Become A Duty To Die:**
Opponents claim that if we are given the legal right to decide the time, place, and manner of our own death, many people will be pressured by family, friends, government, health-care providers, social workers, and/or other patients to exercise that right against their will.

While it is possible that untoward pressure will be applied to a dying relative, the will to live is enormously strong. While the dying person may lovingly consider a survivor's well being, it is more likely that the pain, indignities, and loss of control resulting from the dying process will be the motivation for requesting help in dying. Self interest will normally prevail.

But special care must be made for the abnormal, and for deviant aspects of human nature. The authors of the DDA have considered this possibility and limited those who can help another person die to a licensed physician, and to others under their (i.e., the physician's) control.

If a greedy relative wants a dying loved one out of the way sooner, for instance, he or she would be required to conspire and convince a treating physician that the dying person's life should be ended for reasons not involving the terminal illness or the patient's free will but for other malicious reasons.

The principal check on this kind of abuse is obviously the presence of a doctor and medical team. The dying patient's request must be well considered and enduring. If the physician thinks it is not, he will not provide the requested assistance. His or her response would be something like this: "George, it's true your prognosis is poor, but you're not in pain and your son, who you admit has rarely seen you in the past 20 years, seems inappropriately pressuring you, and I don't want to be a part of that. I'll do what you ask me if it's really your independent request, but I don't believe that is the case here."

If pressure is applied to patients to end their lives, those persons pressuring their dying relative, friend, or ward should be prosecuted for aiding, abetting, and advocating a suicide, which is now a crime in every state in the union. Advocating and encouraging a suicide remains a crime under the DDA.

4. The Patient/Physician Relationship Will Be Weakened:

Critics also claim that if a physician is given the right to end a patient's life upon request, the patient will lose trust in the doctor. Some critics have even suggested that people in rest homes will be afraid to drink whatever liquids they are offered for fear they are poisoned.

This claim is far fetched, but it deserves attention. We must be vigilant and careful of the interests of the most susceptible and weakened members of our society. We must give them the love, care, attention, and treatment that they deserve. We must constantly guard against any abuses of their rights as human beings.

The physician's efforts to preserve our life will ultimately fail in all cases. We will all die regardless of the most aggressive and skilled medical management. The miracles of modern medical science will not make us immortal.

Patients, many of them facing the indignities of a degenerative dying, are now being forced to continue a mere biological existence. Yet surely the patient's respect for the physician will only be enhanced if they and their doctors can plan together for a safe, painless, gentle, timely and dignified death.

Under present law the physician must say, "I'm sorry, I can't help except to keep you alive as long as I can." Honesty between physician and patient and the knowledge that the physician will relieve the horrible pain and suffering associated with many terminal illnesses (when requested) will in fact strengthen the patient/physician relationship and create greater confidence.

Dr. Christiaan Barnard, who performed the first human heart transplant, has stated: "I believe that legalizing euthanasia with controls, would do more to improve the overall quality of American medical care than any other single act."[20] Barnard went on to point out both the sensibleness of a new approach and the difficulty of achieving it: In several European countries, physicians wielded a power that would shock many Americans: the right of active euthanasia.

Dr. Barnard asserts that when a patient in France or in Holland cannot be saved or will be forced to endure a life that is not worth living, doctors need not merely hope that nature will quickly end the ordeal. They can give the hopelessly ill a painless release from suffering. "I believe," continues Barnard "that American medicine would serve people far better if its practitioners also could exercise this mercy. When there is hope of recovery, we must do all that we can to bring it about. But there is no point in using medical technology to prolong a painful death or an empty life. This recognition is causing a fundamental change in medicine, a reordering of its priorities, perhaps like none in history. I believe that eventually this transformation will

---

[20]December 21, 1987 *Omni Magazine*

result in better and more care for the sick. Yet, this revolution will not be easy to bring about, for it requires decisions that violate traditional medicine ethics."[21]

Dr. Barnard argues that simply saving life and prolonging it for years is an improper goal of medicine. The question for medicine today should be whether or not the healing arts provide a meaningful existence so the patient is better off after the treatment than before. By tradition, we venerate length of life, but we must now learn to value quality of life instead.

Patients understand this better than doctors. Patients seldom are obsessed with surviving at all costs, and they grow less so in proportion to the severity of their illness. Most American doctors still feel compelled to treat those they can neither save nor comfort. Dr. Barnard argues that the true goal of medicine should be improving and extending the quality of life, not merely extending biological longevity.

5. **Physicians Should Not Be Executioners:**

Our more strident opponents say that doctors should not kill their patients. They should not be executioners. "Get someone else to do the dirty job," they say.

Our reply is direct. The merciful ending of suffering at life's end upon a patient's request is not killing. Killing implies the ending of a life of someone who wants to live and does not want to die. The man on the gallows, or in the electric chair or gas chamber wants to live; the person who ends the condemned criminal's life is an executioner.

Complying with a terminally ill patient's request for release from the agonies of the final dying process, however, is not killing in the ordinary sense of the word. It is an act of mercy. The disease or the trauma is the killer, not the caring physician who releases his or her patient from their suffering. To suggest that this compassionate act of a physician makes him an executioner and killer is an abuse and misuse of terms.

---

[21]Ibid.

Only physicians have the knowledge that is needed to help us at life's end. The merciful application of their knowledge upon request is totally appropriate. Eighty percent (80%) of Americans die today in some kind of healthcare facility and under a doctor's control and management. Because of the doctor's knowledge, license, and proximity to us at life's end and because merciful release on request is not killing, physicians are the appropriate helping agents.

6. A New Law Is Unnecessary:

Our opponents claim that it is possible to control pain associated with terminal illness in 95% of the cases. They claim that all that is needed is to teach doctors not to worry about making addicts of dying people. They claim that if physicians would only learn to administer sufficient pain-controlling drugs, patients would never suffer. Therefore, ending life to avoid suffering isn't necessary or appropriate.

We reply by denying the assertion that pain can be controlled. Pain cannot be controlled in many cases. According to anesthesiologist, John Dillon, M.D., Professor Emeritus, UCLA Medical School, retired, and others, there are many terminal illnesses where pain simply cannot be abated.

However, even if it were true that pain could be controlled 95% of the time, the other 5% deserve consideration. Moreover, many of those in the purported 95% do not wish to live the final days, weeks, or months of their lives in a stuporous state with little or no cognition or bodily control as a result of massive doses of analgesics, sedatives or anesthetics administered.

Terminally ill persons, irrespective of which "percentage" they fall into, should have the right to make their own decisions about their own life. If it is important to them to retain personal dignity and self-control, they should not be compelled to be dependent on others for every menial function at life's end. They should have the freedom to choose the time and place of their own dying when death is near and certain, and when all treatment options have been exhausted.

7. Euthanasia Is Being Abused in Holland

Dr. Gary F. Krieger, the President of the Los Angeles County Medical Association, claims abuses are occurring in Holland. He claims that some terminal old people and children are being put to death against their will.

There is no significant evidence to support Dr. Krieger's claim. According to Mr. Peter Sutorius of Holland, the prominent attorney who has handled the major cases before his country's Supreme Court relating to voluntary euthanasia, this is not occurring nor is such a possibility being planned. The Dutch Department of Health guidelines do deal with dying children, but these are no different from standard practice in the United States in dealing with dying children. Too often there are difficult moral and ethical problems facing health-care professionals and families with brain-dead and anticephalic children or other gross deformities as to make life, as we know it, impossible. For a full discussion of the practice euthanasia in the Netherlands, see Chapter Three.

8. Physicians Who Administer Aid-In-Dying Under the Death with Dignity Act, if Enacted, Will Violate the Hippocratic Oath:

The full text of the Hippocratic Oath provides as follows:

> I swear by Apollo the physician, by Aesculapius, Hygeia, and Panacea, and I take to witness all of the gods, all the goddesses, to keep according to my ability and my judgment the following Oath: To consider dear to me as my parents him who taught me this art; to live in common with him and if necessary to share my goods with him; to look upon his children as my own brothers, to teach them this art if they so desire without fee or written promise; to impart to my sons and the sons of the master who taught me and the disciples who taught me and the disciples who have enrolled themselves and have agreed to the rules of the profession, but to these alone, the precepts and the instruction. I will prescribe regimen for the good of my patients according to my ability and my judgment and never do

harm to anyone. To please no one will I prescribe a deadly drug, nor give advice which may cause his death. Nor will I give a woman a pessary to procure abortion. But I will preserve the purity even for patients in whom the disease is manifest; I will leave this operation to be performed by practitioners (specialists in this art). In every house where I come I will enter only for the good of my patients, keeping myself far from all intentional ill-doing and all seduction, and especially from the pleasures of love with women or with men, be they free or slaves. All that may come to my knowledge in the exercise of my professions or outside of my profession or in daily commerce with men, which ought not to be spread abroad, I will keep secret and will never reveal. If I keep this oath faithfully, may I enjoy my life and practice my art, respected by all men and in all times; but if I swerve from it or violate it, may the reverse be my lot.

Few, if any, physicians believe in the Greek gods, nor do they swear by Apollo, Aesculapius, Hygeia, and Panacea. To many Catholic, Protestant, and Jewish physicians, taking such an oath to Greek gods would be anathema. In fact, many doctors claim that they have never taken the oath, and that it is not routinely administered by medical schools or by state licensing authorities. True, it is recited at some graduation ceremonies, but the oath is studied by medical students primarily as a part of medical history and medical tradition.

Nevertheless, the oath has served as a reminder to those practicing the healing arts of their obligation to patients and their corresponding duty to sublimate their own good and passion to the concern of patients. The essential provision of the oath is the following:

> I will prescribe regimen for the good of my patients according to my ability and my judgment and will never do harm to anyone.

The oath has not remained inviolate and sacrosanct throughout the years. One of its prescriptions provides: "Nor will I give a woman a pessary to procure an abortion."

Yet, most physicians in this country now agree with freedom of choice for the pregnant woman in some circumstances, demonstrating that the medical profession has not blindly followed the dictates of the oath, but instead applied common sense and modern understanding in a way which violates the oath's literal terms.

Indeed, if Hippocrates were alive today and could see the extent of medical technology—the pumps, tubes, syringes, dialysis machines, respirators, and a myriad of drugs controlling every life function—he probably would have worded his oath differently to accommodate this reality. The oath is nearly 2,500 years old. It was written to deal with its own time.

Helping a dying patient over the final abyss to avoid agony and pain of a final disease is not *harm*. It is mercy. Therefore, even the literal terms of the oath are not violated by the DDA.

9. Legalizing Physician Aid-In-Dying Is the First Step on a Slippery Slope

Some further discussion of the "slippery slope" is needed before criticism can be adequately addressed. According to Indian folklore and history, when an aged squaw became decrepit and could not keep up, and was more of a liability than an asset, she was left along the trail to die. Today, in both Western and Oriental societies, the old are treated differently, largely because of our compassion and because of our society's far greater resources.

Still, critics fear that we will abandon this compassion; they predict that we will allocate resources in other directions and that we will prevent dying individuals who are most often but not always old from deciding for themselves the time and place of their own death, letting someone else make that decision for them. What they fail to recognize is that the allocation of medical resources in America now consumes 11% of gross national product both here and in other advanced societies, and that there are sufficient resources to maintain the health of our older citizens. The allocation of resources for the aged is an important issue, but it is not relevant to this debate.

Permitting me to request and receive physician assistance in dying is totally different from someone else requesting that I die. No one else should control my destiny at life's end absent my instruction and consent, which is a universal proposition applicable to every human being. If someone else decides that my life must end, it is wrong, and in every society it is a crime.

Men and women of ordinary conscience easily make this distinction daily. Moving beyond individual freedom of choice at life's end to eliminating the unwanted and unneeded citizen would be a gross abuse in any civilized society. We must take care to make the distinction, but that requirement should not prevent us from making needed legal change.

10. **We May Become Nazi Germany if We Adopt the Death with Dignity Act**

Dr. Gary F. Krieger, President of the Los Angeles County Medical Association, publicly suggested on two television interviews that we run the risk of becoming a violent and uncaring nation if we adopt the DDA. He pointed out that euthanasia was permitted in Nazi Germany initially, but escalated into mass genocide.

Answering this criticism is hardly necessary because the so-called Nazi "euthanasia" program had nothing to do with mercy, terminal illness, or requested death; rather it was outright murder of the helpless and vulnerable. Also, it is apparent to nearly everyone that Americans are not Nazis. America is not Nazi Germany.

This is not to say we should be complacent, and not be diligent and careful that our government follows the rules and not violate basic sanctions as occurred in Nazi Germany. If a government decides that someone must die, other than for conviction of a capital crime under due process of law, or if a family member decides that another member of the family must die, or if a health-care provider decides that another person must die, that is wrong, it is murder, and the perpetrators must be prosecuted or the government disenfranchised.

Under the DDA, the decision is individual action by an autonomous person about his or her own life, and no one else's life. Freedom to choose the time and place of your own death is a part of the inalienable right of self determination. Enacting the DDA will not lead our country to the atrocities of a Nazi Germany. But taking another's life against their will would make us like Nazi Germany, and that must be avoided at all cost.

That is a major but simple distinction. Advocating a suicide is a crime under the present law in every American state. It will remain a crime after enactment of the DDA. The Act proposes to amend criminal codes so that death resulting from a request for aid-in-dying will not constitute a suicide, and as mentioned, health care professionals and facilities are protected from liability when the patient's wishes are carried out in accordance with the Act.

Specific Objections to the Death with Dignity Act

The following are technical objections to the language of the DDA: 1) the law is not limited to persons in intractable pain, 2) it is not limited to conditions where all treatment options have been exhausted, 3) physicians cannot determine whether or not death will occur within six months, 4) surrogate decision-making is inappropriate and subject to abuse, and 5) the law does not apply to quadriplegic or to persons in a persistive vegetative state who are either not terminal or have not signed a DDA directive. These objections are explained and a full response given in the order listed.

1. **The Law Is Not Limited To Persons In Intractable Pain:**
Professor Alexander Capron, an ethicist who teaches at the University of Southern California Law School and

Medical School in Los Angeles, has publicly observed that the DDA should be restricted to persons in intractable pain.

His criticisms miss the point. Although many dying people wish to end their existence because of intractable pain, many others want to end their lives because of the indignities of the dying process and loss of control. Terminally ill people who are unable to control any of their bodily functions such as bladder, bowels, saliva, or who cannot move their limbs, or who cannot speak or who are totally dependent upon others for every facet of their existence, should have the same rights as those persons in intractable pain. Their right to self-determination is of equal importance.

2. The Law Is Not Limited To Cases Where All Treatment Options Have Been Exhausted.

Professor Capron also complains that the DDA is not explicitly limited to cases where all "treatment options have been exhausted."

Again, Professor Capron misses the point. The DDA is inapplicable unless two physicians have declared the patient to be in a terminal condition. "Terminal condition" is defines in the DDA: "Terminal condition means an *incurable* or *irreversible condition* which will, in the opinion of two certifying physicians exercising reasonable medical judgment, result in death within six months."

The definition of terminal condition specifically says that it is an *"incurable or irreversible condition."* By definition, there is no available treatment option. The patient's condition is incurable, and all treatment options have been exhausted.

3. Physicians Cannot Determine Whether or Not Death Will Occur in Six Months.

Professor Capron and others complain that a physician's prognosis is always imprecise. They claim that it is impossible for any physician to determine that a given patient will die within 180 days. They cite cases where the doctor has predicted six months to live, but the patient survives for years.

Keeping this in mind, the DDA does not require that a physician determine with absolute certainty that death will occur on or before the 180th day. However, it does require that two physicians conclude *with reasonable medical judgment* that death will occur within 180 days or less. That standard is realistic given the current diagnostic and prognostic ability of the medical profession today. Although there are cases where early death is predicted and the patient lives on for years, the fact is that the conclusion of the two physicians that death will occur shortly is usually correct.

Under the DDA, the patient must recognize and assume responsibility for such uncertainty, and for the possibility of physician error. Like all others, physician judgment is fallible, yet knowing and acknowledging this fact, the patient nevertheless undertakes to proceed with or withdraw his or her request for physician aid-in-dying.

4. **Surrogate Decision-Making Is Inappropriate:**

Professor Vickie Michel, of the Loyola University School of Law in Los Angeles and a member of the Los Angeles Bar Association Bioethics Committee, fears that abuses will result if a surrogate decision-maker is permitted because the dying person might change his or her mind while competent but failed to notify anyone of that change of mind. Since a change of mind is a possibility, Professor Michel argues that the request for dying should be limited to only those persons who can have a face-to-face conversation with his or her physician.

Many dying people, perhaps most, would be excluded from the operation of the DDA if the surrogate decision-maker concept were eliminated. Alzheimer's victims, AIDS victims, and others who become incompetent after signing the Directive, would not have their wishes carried out because the terminal condition often does not occur until after the patient is incompetent.

After incompetency, neither a meaningful nor a legal face-to-face patient/physician conversation can occur. Since the number of persons suffering from Alzheimer's disease is increasing throughout the country at an enormous rate, far in excess of the AIDS epidemic, the provision for a surrogate decision-maker is not only appropriate, but imperative. Most courts throughout the country have validated the concept of "substituted judgment" by a surrogate decision-maker. Several of these cases are discussed in Chapter Two.

The DDA provides for revocation by numerous means described in Chapter 4. Moreover, there is an added safeguard of a review by an ethics committee, when a decision is made by an attorney-in-fact.

Section 2525.10 of the DDA provides:

> (a) The decision of an attorney-in-fact to request a physician to administer aid-in-dying shall first be reviewed by a hospital committee of three persons to assure all of the following:
> (1) The directive was properly executed and witnessed.
> (2) The directive has not been revoked by the patient.
> (3) The physicians have certified the patient is terminal.
> (4) The time of death is properly decided by the attorney-in-fact and the physician.
> (b) In reviewing the decision a majority of the committee shall control.
> (c) If the declarant is in a hospital, the three-person committee shall be the ethics committee of that hospital, or three members thereof, or if that hospital does not have an ethics committee, any three persons appointed by the hospital administrator. If the declarant is not in a hospital, the committee shall be selected by the attending physician, and consist of three persons from a hospital ethics committee of a hospital with which the attending physician is affiliated, or three reputable physicians.

5. **The DDA Does Not Go Far Enough Because It Does Not Apply To Quadriplegics or to Persons in a Persistive Vegetative State Who Are Not Terminal and Have Not Signed An DDA Directive:**

Beverly Hills attorney Richard Scott, an Advisory Board member of Americans Against Human Suffering, an advocate of the DDA, and a leading attorney in California on right-to-die issues, observes that the DDA would not apply to persons like Elizabeth Bouvia, the quadriplegic who was the successful litigant in several major appellate decisions in California in 1984, 1986, and 1987. Neither will the DDA apply to Ken, portrayed by actor Richard Dreyfuss in "Whose Life Is It Anyway?" Neither Ken nor Elizabeth was in a terminal condition. Scott asserts that they are entitled to a physician's help in dying even though they are not terminal. Still, society must and does draw lines, extending its sanctions and exemptions to some but not all. Limiting euthanasia to the terminally ill is a reasonable limitation. It is a reasonable line to draw, if not totally logical.

Chapter Six
Our Attempt At Changing The Law: The Task Ahead

Prelude to Change: Options

There is no legal right to die in the United States today other than by withholding or withdrawing artificial life-sustaining devices. As already explained, such an all-inclusive right should exist and the creation of that right with safeguards is the aim of AAHS. Legislative inaction is inexcusable in the face of repeated nudgings from the courts, and in the face of consistent polling data indicating that a clear majority of citizens wish doctor assistance-in-dying when facing a difficult terminal illness.

We argue that the right of freedom of choice is part of the bedrock upon which our democratic society is founded, provided it is responsibly exercised with due regard to the protection of the rights of others. Our United States Constitution was created, in part, to "promote the general welfare and secure the blessings of liberty to ourselves and our posterity." Our Declaration of Independence lists among the inalienable rights endowed upon us by our Creator, "life, liberty, and the pursuit of happiness."

Creating or changing law generally involves the political process. In an ideal political world, a proposed new law affecting every human being in the state, supported by two-thirds of the electorate, and which has been approved and endorsed by the State Bar Association, could get a hearing in the State's legislature.

Ideally, the new measure would be fully aired, with the

arguments of proponents and opponents weighed and considered by the appropriate legislative committee. Special interest groups such as associations of doctors, hospitals, nurses and convalescent hospitals, would explain to the legislative committees how the proposed statute as drafted would affect them. Amendments would be considered by the committee, and its recommendation would be submitted to the legislature. The entire body would consider how the proposed law would affect society as a whole, and then it would either accept or reject it. And ideally, the Governor would then make the same weighty decision and either sign or veto the legislation.

Yet every student of political science knows that changing the law through the legislative process is long, tedious and expensive. It involves locating a legislative sponsor, drafting the legislation in proper statutory language, lobbying the assigned committees to review the legislation in order to motivate them to achieve a majority committee vote in its favor. It involves avoiding debilitating amendments and then repeating the process in the non-originating house. Finally, it involves actively lobbying the Governor to avoid a veto.

Students of political science know that significant numbers of laws are enacted in this fashion every year in state governments all over the country. Yet only those with practical experience know that changing a controversial law or enacting a new concept, even if the new concept is favored by a majority of citizens, is fraught with difficulties because legislatures are largely controlled by vocal minorities and well-financed special interests. The concept of physician aid-in-dying for the terminally ill is both new and controversial and opposed by vocal well-financed minorities.

Why do we struggle to advance the concept of physician aid-in-dying for the terminally ill when there is no similar law anywhere in the Western world, where the opposition is strong and the odds of success are poor? We do so because the cause is worthy, and because two-thirds of the citizens agree with the concept. We hope that an initial breakthrough will come through citizen action via the initiative process. We do so because the initiative process provides a way to sidestep legislatures where special interest groups and vocal or well-finances minorities are largely in control.

The initiative process exists in nearly one-third of the American states. It permits citizens who are registered voters to place measures on the ballot in statewide general elections in order to enact statutes or to amend their constitutions. All states with the initiative process permit constitutional amendments, and all require a greater number of registered voters' signatures on the petitions for ballot qualification than that required to enact a statute. A statute can be placed on the ballot by obtaining signatures of registered voters equalling 5% of those who voted in the last gubernatorial election. Citizen action initiatives and referendums have been legally available in some states for about 75 years. Our hope is that once the DDA is adopted in one or two states by initiative, legislators in the remaining states can thereafter be persuaded to adopt it.

One of the great American ideals is that ours "is a country of laws, not of men." But ours is also a country where legal change is slow, tedious and difficult. Significant changes rarely occur unless there is a major upheaval such as war, revolution, or depression. Although it is not generally recognized, there is just such a major upheaval in our society today. It is prompted by the double-edged advances of medical science and technology, and the delivery of healthcare services which dramatically affect us. It is prompted by many who have seen indignities inflicted on dying loved ones, especially at life's end.

Increasing citizen dissatisfaction is the driving force for legal change permitting freedom of choice at life's end, and permitting terminally ill patients the right to request and receive physician-aid-in-dying. It is also prompted by television and print journalists and by television documentaries. Stories about those who want to die are dramatic, relevant and compelling to viewers and readers.

Efforts, Past and Present

As mentioned in the introduction, the earliest efforts to change the law to permit terminally ill persons this right started on two separate fronts. The first began when Derek Humphry formed the Hemlock Society in 1980 to advance the right of a dying person to active voluntary euthanasia. Mr. Humphry's primary efforts were largely educational, and were advanced through the publication of newsletters, journals and books. He also engaged in television and radio debates with ethicists, physicians and lawyers throughout the country for years. During this initial period, he was essentially the sole spokesman advocating voluntary active euthanasia for the terminally ill.

The second took place in 1985, when fellow attorney Michael White and I, independently and unaware of Mr. Humphry, began efforts to modify the California Natural Death Act (Health & Safety Code Numbers 7185 to 7189.5), and the California Durable Power of Attorney for Health Care Decisions Act (California Civil Code Numbers 2500 to 2513). These two laws were combined and enlarged to include the right of the terminally ill competent adult to request and receive physician aid-in-dying. We named the new law "The Humane and Dignified Death Act (DDA)." Within a year, Michael and I began talking to Derek Humphry and Curt Garbesi, a colleague and law professor at Loyola University School of Law. Both Humphry and Garbesi offered valuable drafting suggestions to the DDA.

Subsequently, we petitioned the Beverly Hills Bar Association to sponsor a resolution advocating the DDA before the State Bar of California at its 1986 convention. The Beverly Hills Bar Association Resolution Committee reviewed our draft, made invaluable suggestions and criticisms (most of which were incorporated in a revised version of the original draft), and voted to recommend that the Association sponsor the DDA. The revised DDA was then adopted by the Beverly Hills Bar Board of Governors, who in turn agreed to sponsor the resolution before the State Bar meeting in Monterey in 1986. The resolution was narrowly defeated in 1986, but success was only a year away.

Soon after the resolution was defeated in 1986, we sent copies of the proposed DDA to each of California's 80 assemblymen and 40 senators to ask for their sponsorship, endorsement or help in order to enact the proposed statute. Not a single legislator replied. Although the Board of Delegates of the State Bar of California adopted a resolution similar to the DDA in 1987, I could not find one California legislator who would risk incurring the wrath of his opponents. The Beverly Hills Bar Association's paid lobbyist in Sacramento was similarly unsuccessful in finding even one legislative sponsor.

At about the same time, over 27,000 supporters of Americans Against Human Suffering, Inc. (AAHS) signed petitions to their Congressmen urging adoption of a Congressional resolution, urging those several states to enact the DDA. Yet those petitions did not cause a single U.S. Congressman to sponsor such a resolution before Congress. It became clear that legislators would not deal with this issue. Alternative ways to accomplish our goal were needed, which lead us inevitably to the initiative process. Unfortunately, the initiative process was and is enormously expensive.

We therefore embarked upon a direct mail fund-raising program, hoping to place the DDA on the November 1988 California ballot by the initiative process in the same manner as the famous Proposition 13 tax limitation nearly 14 years ago. A direct mail campaign would also permit us to reach many citizens throughout the country to prepare for the adoption of similar measures in other states. Initial testing of such a campaign proved that like-minded citizens throughout the country would support our effort in California with their hard-earned money. Actor Richard Dreyfuss, who starred in the film, "Whose Life Is It Anyway?" and whose public profile supports a pro-euthanasia stand, helped with our initial appeals by offering a supportive letter.

The first test mailings were followed by two larger mailings in September and in November 1987. The September mailing was disappointing in terms of total dollars received, but encouraging in several other respects. Persons who were not previously connected with the right-to-die movement responded generously. However, difficulties with the one million-piece mailer in November 1987 raised little money, which meant that obtaining the 450,000 registered voters' signatures by mail would be virtually impossible.

Simultaneously, with the direct mail effort, we pursued another method of obtaining the needed signatures by contacting a professional signature-gathering firm, American Petition Consultants (APC), who agreed to begin circulating petitions in mid-December 1987. We had some money earmarked for the professional signature-gathering firm, but not nearly the $350,000 required to assure the initiative's qualification. Obviously, APC would not work without payment, and discontinued their effort in January. It should be noted that no initiative in California has ever qualified without professional signature-gathering services in the last 30 years.

There was one positive side benefit from this campaign. Americans Against Human Suffering, Inc. (AAHS) now has grown to a membership of nearly 30,000 supporting citizens around the country. Most have signed petitions to their representatives urging adoption of a congressional resolution urging the states to pass the DDA.

Fortunately, we had begun a fourth method of qualifying the initiative by seeking volunteers throughout the state to help circulate petitions. Initially, we intended the volunteer effort to supplement the professional signature-gathering effort, but because of lack of money, the burden fell entirely on our unpaid army of workers, the majority of them senior citizens. The enormous effort by innumerable people, particularly in San Diego, Santa Barbara and San Francisco, helped make the initiative front-page and prime-time news, not only in California, but all over the United States. Were it not for this volunteer effort, we would not have obtained the massive publicity given us by the television and print media.

Responses in the medical community have been mixed. Opposition has come from the American Medical Association and its counterparts. However, American medicine is a house divided on this issue. The Los Angeles County Medical Association is typical of associations throughout the country. Despite official disapproval, a survey of its members in the May 1988 issue of its publication, *Physician*, indicated that 40% of the physicians who responded favored the initiative, while 42% favor active euthanasia.

A survey of California physicians conducted by the Hemlock Society in November of 1987 indicated that nearly two-thirds of the physicians who responded believe the law should be changed to allow doctors to take active steps to bring about a patient's death under some circumstances. Fifty-one percent of those responding indicated they would practice active voluntary euthanasia if it were legal.

On May 8, 1988, the *Los Angeles Times* reported a survey conducted by the San Francisco Medical Society of its members. Of the 750 physicians who participated, 75% supported making voluntary euthanasia legal for patients. Forty-five percent said they would carry out such a request from patients.

Recognition and support has come from the mental health community. The Board of Directors of the California State Psychological Association, after a committee study of the DDA, voted to support the Initiative: "In the interests of promoting human welfare, [it] endorsed the general principle of granting to a terminally ill individual the right to request physician aid-in-dying as described in the Humane and Dignified Death Initiative (now the Death with Dignity Act) sponsored by Americans Against Human Suffering, Inc. (AAHS)."[22] In an article reporting the Board's action, Board member May Lee Ziskin, its liaison to Americans Against Human Suffering, reported also on an article by Leo Rangle, M.D., entitled "The Decision to Terminate One's Life: Psychoanalytic Thoughts on Suicide," in *Suicide and Life-*

---

[22]From "The California Psychologist," Vol. XXII, No. 5 (October, 1988).

Suicide today is not proof of psychosis. The problem of irrational or involuntary suicide must be worked through theoretically as clinical life situations become more complex... The right to end one's life, common sense suicide, is seen as the final right... to choose a painless over a tortured painracked death.[23]

Responses of religious groups is also varied. The Catholic Church is opposed to voluntary active euthanasia, but 61% of Catholic parishioners are in favor of the idea according to a Roper Poll conducted in 1988. A few Protestant denominations are opposed, although the issue is often left up to the individual dictates of each minister and parishioner. The Jewish hierarchy is opposed, but Jewish people are in favor by the largest percentage (69%) of any religious denomination. The Humanist Society also supports the initiative.

At its June 1988 International General Assembly, the Unitarian Universalist Association of Congregations passed a resolution which read, in part, that they:

> ...advocate the right of self-determination in dying and the release from civil or criminal penalties of those who, under proper safeguards, act to honor the right of terminally ill patients to select the time of their own deaths...[and that] Unitarian Universalists...inform and petition legislators to support legislation that will create legal protection for the right to die with dignity in accordance with one's own choice.

Clearly we have gained momentum. Membership in the National Hemlock Society, the "think tank" of the voluntary euthanasia movement, has climbed to over 30,000. The Society's motto is "Good Life. Good Death," based on proper translation from the Greek of our word, euthanasia. Membership in Americans Against Human Suffering has reached over 30,000 in the short space of two years. Support from professional associations has begun to climb. Among

---

[23]Dr. Rangle is clinical professor of psychiatry at the University of California at Los Angeles and San Francisco.

individual professionals in a variety of disciplines, the climb has been dramatic.

Lay, religious, professional and governmental groups are beginning to study carefully the problems not only of those who are going but those who are approaching death. There is a growing credence in what many of the dying have been saying for a long time, "Let me die in peace. Let me escape pain and suffering! Let me conserve my resources to be used for the benefit of posterity rather than squandered on ultimately useless medical procedures. Let me die with dignity!"

Support from the media has been nothing short of spectacular. Professionals among them have recognized the validity of the issues involved over the right-to-die. Equally seen are roles played by patients wishing to express their autonomy and doctors, too many of whom are more concerned with fighting diseases than in treating patients as thinking and feeling people.

These issues entail high drama. They are newsworthy. They are worthy of thoughtful consideration, evoking rational analysis, identifying of alternatives, and synthesis into public policy agreements about what shall be done. But there is also evidence of the clash between cultural differences and the heavy hands of custom and tradition on the one hand and new realities in dying and needs for beneficial change to meet them on the other. Where are we heading?

Our Task Ahead

Our task is to bring about what appears to us and many others a much wanted and beneficial change in public policy as expressed in law. It is to enact the Death with Dignity Act, or some close approximation thereof.

AAHS now plans to qualify the Death with Dignity Act (DDA) by initiative in California for the November 1992 general election. This time, AAHS hopes to have the money needed to pay professional signature-gatherers and hopes to have a well-organized corp of volunteers to begin as soon as is legally possible to gather those signatures. In California, the required number of signatures must be gathered within 150 days after the State Attorney General's Office issues a title and summary of the initiative.

In summary, AAHS plans to move forward aggressively on several fronts.

- Seek legislative sponsors for the DDA in states where the initiative procedure is unavailable;
- Circulate petitions in five or six states with the initiative process in 1992 (states other than Oregon and Washington);
- Establish AAHS affiliates or task forces in every major U.S. city;
- Continue to raise money through direct mail and expand our donor base, as well as develop plans for fundraising events initially in California;
- Contract with an established effective and reputable campaign manager to run a media campaign after qualification in Oregon and California;
- Contract with a professional signature-gathering firm to supplement and augment our volunteer signature-gatherers;
- Determine the feasibility of pursuing an initiative campaign process in the state of Florida and in California for 1992.

Needless to say, help is needed on all fronts to accomplish these tasks. We need chapters organized in each community. We need people willing to take the lead in this chapter formation. We need speakers, writers, secretaries, and signature-gatherers when the time comes. We need specific sites for the distribution of petitions to persons willing to obtain signatures. Most urgently, we need money to hire professional signature-gatherers.

Finally, we'll need a well-conceived media campaign to properly carry the message in anticipation of criticism following qualification of the initiative. Success will require sacrifice of time, talent and money of thousands of socially-conscious, concerned Americans. We will do it together. The wishes of nearly two-thirds of the population mandates enactment of the DDA. Our time has come.

Ours will be a political campaign of no small order. We

hope that you, the reader of this book, will volunteer your ideas, talent, time and hard-earned funds to make it successful. We hope that you will find the cause worth fighting for. We hope that we can achieve, perhaps for ourselves and for some at least, an easier dying process. Surely this is worth an effort on your part. Whatever contribution you may make to this cause may be considered a down payment on the right to choose a "good death."

If the law is changed, it will be *you* who will be in charge of the circumstances of your dying. That's why the enactment of the Death with Dignity Act is so important.

Conclusion

Millions of us will approach life's end, no longer able to bear the pain because of the deterioration of the body and the distressed quality of life from cancer, AIDS, or other illness. We may wish to decide to end the pain and suffering at the time and place of our choice. We should be permitted this choice under law since our self-determination is the most basic of freedoms and is constitutionally protected. Self-determination includes the absolute right to control our own goals and values as long as they do not infringe upon the rights of others. These rights ought to include our right to die at life's end at the time and place of our choosing, whether by active or passive means with the help of the medical profession.

The Death with Dignity Act does so provide.

Simply stated, the Act permits an adult the right to request and receive a physician's aid-in-dying under carefully defined circumstances. It immunizes and protects physicians and health-care workers from liability in carrying out the patient's wishes. To take advantage of this law, a competent adult person must sign the Death with Dignity Act (DDA) directive, which is specified in the statute.

Appendix A

A Proposal
The California Death With Dignity Act
California Civil Code, Title 10.5

SEC. 1. Title 10.5 (commencing with Section 2525) is added to Division 3 of Part 4 of the Civil Code, to read:

2525. This title shall be known and may be cited as the Death With Dignity Act.

2525.1. Self-determination is the most basic of freedoms. The right to die at the time and place of our own choosing when we are terminally ill is an integral part of our right to control our own destinies. That right should be established in law but limited to ensure that the rights of others are not affected. The right should include the ability to make a conscious and informed choice to enlist the help of the medical profession in making death as painless and quick as possible.

Adult persons have the fundamental right to control the decisions relating to the rendering of their own medical care, including the decisions to have life-sustaining procedures withheld or withdrawn or when suffering from a terminal condition, as defined herein, to request a physician to administer aid-in-dying.

Modern medical technology has made possible the artificial prolongation of human life beyond natural limits. This prolongation of life for persons with terminal conditions may cause loss of patient dignity and unnecessary pain and suffering, while providing nothing medically necessary or beneficial to the patient.

In recognition of the dignity and privacy which patients have a right to expect, the State of California shall recognize the right of an adult terminally ill person to make a written directive instructing his or her physician to administer aid-in-dying or to withhold or withdraw life-sustaining procedures.

The purpose of this Act is to create a legal right to request and receive physician aid-in-dying, and to protect and exonerate physicians who voluntarily comply with the request. No one is required to take advantage of this legal right or participate if they are morally or ethically opposed.

2525.2. The following definitions shall govern the construction of this title:

>   (a) "Attending physician" means the physician selected by, or assigned to, the patient and who has primary responsibility for the treatment and care of the patient.
>   (b) "Directive" means a written document and Durable Power of Attorney voluntarily executed by the declarant in accordance with the requirements of Section 2525.3 in the form set forth in Section 2526.5.
>   (c) "Declarant" means a person who executes a directive, in accordance with this title.
>   (d) "Life-sustaining procedure" means any medical procedure or intervention which utilizes mechanical or other artificial means to sustain, restore, or supplant a vital function, including nourishment and hydration which, when applied to a qualified patient, would serve only artificially to prolong the moment of death. "Life-sustaining procedure" shall not include the administration of medication or the performance of any medical procedure deemed necessary to alleviate pain.

(e) "Physician" means a physician and surgeon licensed by the Board of Medical Quality Assurance or the Board of Osteopathic Examiners.

(f) "Qualified patient" means an adult patient who has executed a directive as defined in this section, which directive is currently valid, who is suffering and has been diagnosed and certified in writing by two physicians to be afflicted with a terminal condition. One of said physicians shall be the attending physician, who has personally examined the patient.

(g) "Terminal condition" means an incurable or irreversible condition which will in the opinion of two certifying physicians exercising reasonable medical judgment result in death within six months.

(h) "Aid-in-dying" means any medical procedure that will terminate the life of the qualified patient swiftly, painlessly, and humanely.

(i) "Attorney-in-fact" means an agent of the person or patient signing the directive, appointed for the purpose of making decisions relating to the patient's medical care and treatment, including withdrawal of life-sustaining procedures and physician aid-in-dying, in the event the patient becomes incompetent to make those decisions. An attorney-in-fact shall be an adult, who may, but need not, be related to the person or patient, but an attorney-in-fact need not be an attorney at law or a lawyer.

(j) "Health-care provider" means a person licensed, certified, or otherwise authorized by the law of this state to administer health care in the ordinary course of business or practice of a profession.

2525.3. An adult individual of sound mind may at any time execute a directive governing the withholding or withdrawal of life-sustaining procedures or administering aid-in-dying and appoint an attorney-in-fact. The directive shall be signed by the declarant and witnessed by two individuals, not related to the declarant by blood or marriage and who would not be entitled to any portion of the estate of the declarant upon his/her death under any will of the declarant or codicil thereto then existing, or, at the time of the directive, by operation of law then existing. In addition, a witness to a directive shall not be the attending physician, an employee of the attending physician who is involved in any way with the treatment of the individual, or an employee of a health care facility in which the declarant is a patient, or any person who, at the time of the execution of the directive, has a claim against any portion of the estate of the declarant upon his or her death. The directive shall be in the form contained in Section 2526.

2525.4. A directive shall have no force or effect if the declarant is a patient in a skilled nursing facility as defined in subdivision (c) or Section 1250 of the Health and Safety Code and intermediate care facilities or community care facilities at the time the directive is executed unless one of the two witnesses to the directive is a patient advocate or ombudsman designated by the Department of Aging for this purpose pursuant to any other applicable provision of law. The patient advocate or ombudsman shall have the same qualifications as a witness under Section 2525.3.

The intent of this section is to recognize that some patients in skilled nursing facilities may be so insulated from a voluntary decision-making role, by virtue of the custodial nature of their care, as to require special assurance that they are capable of willfully and voluntarily executing a directive.

2525.5. (a) A directive may be revoked at any time by the declarant, without regard to his or her mental state or competency, by any of the following methods:

(1) By being canceled, defaced, obliterated, or burned, torn, or otherwise destroyed by the and at the direction of the declarant with the intent to revoke the directive.

(2) By a written revocation of the declarant expressing his or her intent to revoke the directive, signed and dated by the declarant. This revocation shall become effective only upon communication to the attending physician by the declarant or by a person acting on behalf of the declarant. The attending physician shall record in the patient's medical record the time and date when he or she received notification of the written revocation, and the identity of the communicator.

(3) By a verbal expression by the declarant of his or her intent to revoke the directive. The revocation shall become effective only upon communication to the attending physician by the declarant or by a person acting on behalf of the declarant. The attending physician shall confirm with the patient that he or she wishes to revoke and shall record in the patient's medical record the time, date, and place of the revocation and the time, date, and place, if different, that he or she received notification of the revocation, and the identity of the notifier.

(b) There shall be no criminal, civil, or administrative liability on the part of any person for following a directive that has been revoked unless that person has actual knowledge of the revocation.

2525.6. (a) Except as provided in subdivision (b), a directive shall be effective for seven years from the date of execution thereof unless revoked prior to the end of the seven-year time period in the manner prescribed in Section 2525.5. This title shall not prevent a declarant from re-executing a directive at any time in accordance with Section 2525.3, including re-execution subsequent to a diagnosis of a terminal condition. If the declarant has executed more than one directive, the seven-year time period specified in this section shall be deemed to commence on the date of execution of the last directive known to the attending physician.

(b) If the declarant becomes comatose or is otherwise rendered incapable of communicating with the attending physician before the end of the seven-year period, the directive shall remain in effect for the duration of the comatose condition or until such time as the declarant's condition renders him or her able to communicate with the attending physician.

2525.7. No physician or employee of a health care facility who, acting in accordance with the requirements of this title, causes the withholding or withdrawal of life-sustaining procedures from, or administers aid-in-dying to, a qualified patient, shall be subject to civil, criminal, or administrative liability therefore. No licensed health care professional, such as a nurse, acting under the direction of a physician, who participates in the withholding or withdrawal of life-sustaining procedures from, or administers aid-in-dying to, a qualified patient in accordance with this title shall be subject to any civil, criminal, or administrative liability. No physician, or other person acting under the direction of a physician, who acts in accordance with the provisions of this chapter, shall be guilty of any criminal act or of unprofessional conduct because he or she participates in the withholding or withdrawal of life-sustaining procedures, or because he or she administers aid-in-dying. Fees for administering aid-in-dying shall be fair and reasonable.

> (a) The certifying physicians shall not be partners or shareholders in the same practice.

2525.8. (a) Nothing herein requires a physician or licensed health professional, such as nurses, to administer aid-in-dying if he or she is morally or ethically opposed. Neither shall privately owned hospitals be required to permit the administration of physician aid-in-dying in their facilities if they are morally and ethically opposed.

(b) With the consent of a qualified patient, the attending physician who is requested to give aid-in-dying may request a psychiatric or psychological consultation if said physician has any question about the patient's competence.

2525.9. (a) Prior to withholding or withdrawing life-sustaining procedures from, or administering aid-in-dying to, a qualified patient pursuant to a directive, the attending physician shall determine that the directive complies with Section 2525.3, and that the directive and all steps proposed by the attending physician to be undertaken are in accord with the desires of the qualified patient, as expressed in the directive.

(b) If the declarant is a qualified patient, the directive shall be conclusively presumed, unless revoked, to be the directions of the patient regarding the withholding or withdrawal of life-sustaining procedures. No physician, and no person acting under the direction of a physician, shall be criminally, civilly, or administratively liable for failing to effectuate the directive of the qualified patient, unless he willfully fails to transfer the patient upon request.

2525.10 (a) The decision of an attorney-in-fact to request a physician to administer aid-in-dying shall first be reviewed by a hospital committee of three persons to assure all of the following:
(1) The directive was properly executed and witnessed.
(2) The directive has not been revoked by the patient.
(3) The physicians have certified the patient is terminal.
(4) The time of death is properly decided by the attorney-in-fact and the physician.
(b) In reviewing the decision of an attorney-in-fact, the decision of a majority of the committee shall control.
(c) If the declarant is in a hospital, the three-person committee shall be the ethics committee of that hospital, or three members thereof, or if that hospital does not have an ethics committee, any three persons appointed by the hospital administrator. If the declarant is not in a hospital, the committee shall be selected by the attending physician, and consist of three persons from a hospital ethics committee of a hospital with which the attending physician is affiliated, or three reputable physicians.

2526. (a) The withholding or withdrawal of life-sustaining procedures from, or administering aid-in-dying to, a qualified patient in accordance with this title shall not, for any purpose,

constitute a suicide.
(b) The making of a directive pursuant to Section 2525.3 shall not restrict, inhibit, or impair in any manner the sale, procurement, or issuance of any policy of life or health insurance, nor shall it affect in any way the terms of an existing policy of life or health insurance. No policy of life or health insurance shall be legally impaired or invalidated in any manner by the withholding or withdrawal of life-sustaining procedures from, or administering aid-in-dying to, an insured qualified patient, notwithstanding any term of the policy to the contrary.
(c) No physician, health facility, or other health-care provider, and no health-care service plan, insurer issuing disability insurance, self-insured employee welfare benefit plan, or nonprofit hospital service plan shall require any person to execute a directive as a condition for being insured for, or receiving, health-care services, nor refuse service because of the execution, the existence, or the revocation of a directive.
(d) A person who requires or prohibits the execution of a directive as a condition for being insured for, or receiving, health-care services is guilty of a misdemeanor.
(e) A person who coerces or fraudulently induces another to execute a directive under this chapter is guilty of a misdemeanor, or if death occurs as a result of said fraud or coercion, is guilty of a felony.

2526.1. This title shall not impair or supersede any legal right or legal responsibility which any person may have to effect the withholding or withdrawal of life-sustaining procedures or administering aid-in-dying in any lawful manner.

91

In this respect the provisions of this title are cumulative.

2526.2. Any person who willfully conceals, cancels, defaces, obliterates, or damages the directive of another without the declarant's consent shall be guilty of a misdemeanor. Any person who falsifies or forges the directive of another, or willfully conceals or withholds personal knowledge of a revocation as provided in Section 2525.5, with the intent to cause a withholding or withdrawal of life-sustaining procedures or to induce aid-in-dying procedures contrary to the wishes of the declarant, and thereby, because of such act, directly causes life-sustaining procedures to be withheld or withdrawn and death thereby to be hastened or aid-in-dying to be administered, shall be subject to prosecution for unlawful homicide as provided in Chapter 1 (commencing with Section 187) of Title 8 of Part 1 of the Penal Code.

2526.3. Compliance with a qualified patient's directive pursuant to this title, even if this compliance results in hastening the death of the qualified patient, is not a crime. No person who participates in any manner in the compliance with the directive shall be liable for any civil or administrative damages or penalties because of his or her participation or of the death of the qualified patient.

2526.4. (a) Hospitals and other health-care providers who carry out the directive of a qualified patient shall keep a record of the number of these cases, and report annually to the State Department of Health Services the patient's age, type of illness, and the date the directive was carried out. In all cases, the identity of the patient and the attorney-in-fact shall be strictly confidential and shall not be reported.

(b) The directive, or a copy of the directive, shall be made a part of a patient's medical records in each institution involved in the patient's medical care.

2526.5. In order for a directive to be valid under this title, the directive shall be in the following form:

DIRECTIVE TO PHYSICIANS

Warning to Patient

This is an important legal document. Before executing this document, you should know these important facts:

Powers to Agent

This document gives your agent (the attorney-in-fact) when you are in a coma or otherwise unable to act or decide for yourself:

1. The power to decide the time of your death for you. However, your agent must act consistently with your desires, as stated in this document or otherwise made known to him or her.

2. The power to direct your physician to administer aid-in-dying, if you have been diagnosed by two licensed physicians as terminal.

3. Authority to consent or refuse consent to any treatment, service or procedure for diagnosis or treatment of any physical or mental condition. This power is limited by your desires contained in this statement. You can provide in this document the type of treatment that you desire or do not desire.

4. The right to examine your medical records and consent to their disclosure unless you limit this right in this document.

Duration

The power granted by this document shall exist for seven years from the date it is signed unless you specify a shorter period. If you are unable to decide the appropriateness of instructing your physician to administer aid-in-dying at the time this seven-year period ends, the power will continue to exist until the time you become able to make a decision for yourself or your agent decides to honor the directive.

Revocation

You may revoke the authority of your agent and his or her power by notifying him or her, or your treating physician, hospital, or other health-care provider, orally or in writing.

This document revokes any prior directive to withhold or withdraw life-support systems, or to administer aid-in-dying.

Procedures

You must follow the witnessing procedures described at the end of this form. If you fail to follow the procedures, this document will not be valid.

Your agent may need this document immediately in an emergency. Therefore keep it where it is immediately available to your agent. It is recommended that you give your agent a signed copy. You may also wish to give your doctor a signed copy.

Limitations

The court can take away the power of your agent to make health-care decisions, to act in your behalf, and to direct your physician to administer aid-in-dying if he or she acts contrarily to your known desires.

Do not use this form if you are a conservatee under the Lanterman-Petris-Short Act and you want to appoint your conservator as your agent. You can do that only if the appointment document includes a certificate of your attorney. Nothwithstanding your instructions in this directive, life-support systems may not be withdrawn or withheld when necessary to keep you alive if you or your agent object at the time.

Instructions

This directive is made this _____ day of _____ (month) _____ (year).

I, _____ being of sound mind, willfully and voluntarily make known my desire

    (a) ☐ **That my life shall not be artificially prolonged** and
    (b) ☐ **That my life shall be ended with the aid of a physician under the circumstances set forth below, and do hereby declare:**
    (You must initial (a) or (b), or both.)

1. If at any time I should have a terminal condition or illness certified to be terminal by two physicians, and they determine that my death will occur within six months,

    (a) ☐ **I direct that life-sustaining procedures be withheld or withdrawn,** and

(b) ☐ **I direct that my physician administer aid-in-dying in a humane and dignified manner.** (You must initial (a) or (b), or both.)

(c) ☐ **I have attached Special Instructions on a separate page to the directive.** (Initial if you have attached a separate page.)

The action taken under this paragraph shall be at the time of my own choosing if I am competent.

2. In the absence of my ability to give directions regarding the termination of my life, it is my intention that this directive shall be honored by my family, agent (described in paragraph 5), and physician(s) as the final expression of my legal right to

(a) ☐ **Refuse medical or surgical treatment,** and
(b) ☐ **To choose to die in a humane and dignified manner.** (You must initial (a) or (b), or both and you must initial one box below.)

☐ If I am unable to give directions, I *do not* want my attorney-in-fact to request aid-in-dying.

☐ If I am unable to give directions, I *do* want my attorney-in-fact to ask my physician for aid-in-dying.

3. I understand that a terminal condition is one in which I am not likely to live for more than six months.

4. a. I, _____

do hereby designate and appoint _____

as my attorney-in-fact (agent) to make health-care decisions for me if I am in a coma or otherwise unable to decide for myself as authorized in this document. For the purpose of this document, "health-care decision" means consent, refusal of consent, or withdrawal of consent to any care, treatment, service, or procedure to maintain, diagnose, or treat an individual's physical or mental condition, or to administer aid-in-dying.

b. By this document I intend to create a Durable Power of Attorney for Health Care under The Death with Dignity Act and Sections 2430 to 2443, inclusive, of the Civil Code. This power of attorney shall not be affected by my subsequent incapacity, except by revocation.

c. Subject to any limitations in this document, I hereby grant to my agent full power and authority to make health-care decisions for me to the same extent that I could make these decisions for myself if I had the capacity to do so. In exercising this authority, my agent shall make health-care decisions that are consistent with my desires as stated in this document or otherwise made known to my agent, including, but not limited to, my desires concerning obtaining, refusing, or withdrawing life-prolonging care, treatment, services and procedures, and administration of aid-in-dying.

5. This directive shall have no force or effect seven years from the date filled in above, unless I am incompetent to act on my own behalf and then it shall remain valid until my competency is restored.

6. I recognize that a physician's judgment is not always certain, and that medical science continues to make progress in extending life, but in spite of these facts, I nevertheless wish aid-in-dying rather than letting my terminal condition take its natural course.

7. My family has been informed of my request to die, their opinions have been taken into consideration, but the final decision remains mine, so long as I am competent.

8. The exact time of my death will be determined by me and my physician with my desire or my attorney-in-fact's instructions paramount.

I have given full consideration and understand the full import of this directive, and I am emotionally and mentally competent to make this directive. I accept the moral and legal responsibility for receiving aid-in-dying.

This directive will not be valid unless it is signed by two qualified witnesses who are present when you sign or acknowledge your signature. The witnesses must not be related to you by blood, marriage, or adoption; they must not be entitled to any part of your estate; and they must not include a physician or other person responsible for, or employed by anyone responsible for, your health care. If you have attached any additional pages to this form, you

must date and sign each of the additional pages at the same time you date and sign this power of attorney.

Signed: _____

City, County, and State of Residence

(This document must be witnessed by two qualified adult witnesses. None of the following may be used as witnesses: (1) a health care provider who is involved in any way with the treatment of the declarant, (2) an employee of a health-care provider who is involved in any way with the treatment of the declarant, (3) the operator of a community care facility where the declarant resides, (4) an employee of an operator of a community care facility who is involved in any way with the treatment of the declarant.

I declare under penalty of perjury under the laws of California that the person who signed or acknowledged this document is personally known to me (or proved to me on the basis of satisfactory evidence) to be the declarant of this directive; that he or she signed and acknowledged this directive in my presence, that he or she appears to be of sound mind and under no duress, fraud, or undue influence; that I am not a health-care provider, an employee of a health-care provider, the operator of a community-care facility, nor an employee of an operator of a community-care facility where the declarant resides.

I further declare under penalty of perjury under the laws of California that I am not related to the principal by blood, marriage, or adoption, and, to the best of my knowledge, I am not entitled to any part of the estate of the principal upon the death of the principal under a will now existing or by operation of law.

Date: _____
Witness's Signature: _____
Print Name: _____
Residence Address: _____
Date: _____
Witness's Signature: _____
Print Name: _____
Residence Address: _____

STATEMENT OF PATIENT ADVOCATE OR OMBUDSMAN
(If you are a patient in a skilled nursing facility, one of the witnesses must be a patient advocate or ombudsman. The following statement is required only if you are a patient in a skilled nursing facility—a health-care facility that provides the following basic services: skilled nursing care and supportive care to patients whose primary need is for availability of skilled nursing care on an extended basis. The patient advocate or ombudsman must sign both parts of the "Statement of Witnesses" above AND must also sign the following statement.)

I further declare under penalty of perjury under the laws of California that I am a patient advocate or ombudsman as designated by the State Department of Aging and that I am serving as a witness as required by Section 2525.4 of the California Civil Code.

Signed: _____

2526.6. The fact that a patient is a burden or is incompetent shall not be a factor in any decision to withhold or withdraw life-sustaining procedures, or to administer aid-in-dying.

Sec. 2. Neither the Natural Death Act, California Health and Safety Code Sections 7185-7189.5 nor the Durable Power of Attorney for Health Care, California Civil Code Sections 2500-2513 shall be effected hereby. The sanctions provided in this section do not displace any sanction applicable under other law, except as specifically provided.

Sec. 3. CALIFORNIA CIVIL CODE SECTION 2443. Mercy Killing Not Be Condoned. Nothing in this article shall be construed to condone, authorize, or approve mercy killing, or to permit any affirmative or deliberate act or omission to end life other than the withholding or withdrawal of health-care pursuant to a Durable Power of Attorney for Health Care so as to permit the natural process of dying or enlisting physician aid-in-dying under the provisions of the

Death with Dignity Act, California Civil Code, Title 10.5.

Sec. 4. Section 401 of the Penal Code is amended to read: "401. Every person who deliberately aids, or advises, or encourages another to commit suicide, is guilty of a felony. Death resulting from a request for aid-in-dying or from a withholding or withdrawing of treatment pursuant to Title 10.5 (commencing with Section 2525) of Division 3 of Part 4 of the Civil Code shall not constitute suicide nor is a licensed physician who lawfully administers aid-in-dying or who lawfully withdraws or withholds treatment, or a health-care provider or health professional acting under the direction of a physician, liable under this section. Death resulting from the withholding or withdrawal of a life-sustaining procedure or aid-in-dying pursuant to a directive in accordance with the Death With Dignity Act does not, for any purpose, constitute a suicide or homicide."

Sec. 5. This act may be amended only by a statute passed by a two-thirds vote of each house of the legislature and signed by the Governor.

Sponsored by:
AMERICANS AGAINST HUMAN SUFFERING
P.O. Box 11001
Glendale, CA 91206
818/240-1986

July 1, 1989

Appendix B

The Death with Dignity Act
(What it Does)

Prepared by Robert L. Risley, author of the Death with Dignity Act, formerly the Humane and Dignified Death Act Initiative, and President of Americans Against Humane Suffering.

• Permits a competent terminally ill adult the right to request and receive physician aid-in-dying under carefully defined circumstances.
• Protects physicians from liability in carrying out a patient's request.
• Combines the concepts of Natural Death Acts and Durable Power of Attorney for Health Care laws, and makes them more usable.
• Permits a patient to appoint an attorney-in-fact to make health care decisions, including withholding and withdrawing life-support systems, and can empower the attorney-in-fact to decide about requesting aid-in-dying if the patient becomes incompetent.
• Requires decision of the attorney-in-fact to be reviewed by a hospital ethics or other committee before the decision is acted upon by the physician.
• To take advantage of the law, a competent adult person must sign a Death with Dignity (DDA) directive.
• Permits revocation of a directive at any time by any means.
• Requires hospitals and other health-care facilities to

keep records and report to the Department of Health Services after the death of the patient and then anonymously.

• Permits a treating physician to order a psychiatric consultation, with the patient's consent if there is any question about the patient's competence to make the request for aid-in-dying.

• Forbids aid-in-dying to any patient solely because he/she is a burden to anyone, or because the patient is incompetent or terminal and has not made out an informed and proper (DDA) directive.

• Forbids aiding, abetting, and encouraging a suicide which remains a crime under the Act.

• Does not permit aid-in-dying to be administered by a loved one, family member, or stranger.

• Forbids aid-in-dying for children, incompetents, or anyone who has not voluntarily and intentionally completed and signed the properly witnessed (DDA) directive.

• Attempts to keep the decision-making process with the patient and health-care provider, and out of court.

• Makes special protective provisions for patients in skilled nursing facilities.

• Provides for amendment by a two-thirds vote of the legislature and signature of the Governor.

• Permits doctors, nurses, and privately owned hospitals the right to decline a dying patient's request for aid-in-dying if they are morally or ethically opposed to such action.

Questions and Answers

Q: *Why change the law?*

A: Because there has been a dramatic change in medical technology and the delivery of health-care services in the past fifty years, and the law has not kept pace. For those nearing life's end, there is a new mechanized medical reality not existing fifty years ago. Today dying is often postponed, for which we are grateful, but in some cases it is prolonged against the dying patient's will.

Present law permits patients to direct the withdrawal or

removal of life-support systems for the terminally ill that would result in their death. However, as noted, the law does not provide for those dying of a terminal disease who are not on life-support systems, even though they do not wish to have their dying prolonged. Doctors do increase pain-controlling drugs, which may intentionally or inadvertently cause death, but this is rarely discussed with the patient. It should be discussed and decisions should be made with the patient. It should be discussed and decisions should be made, with the patient being primary decision-maker. As Richard Dreyfuss asked in the film of the same name, "Whose life is it, anyway?"

Q: *Why use the initiative?*
A: Because it is unlikely that legislatures will pass such a law, even though two-thirds of our citizens are in favor to it.

Q: *Who will oppose the act?*
A: We expect many, but not all, religious organizations to oppose the act, even though many individual parishioners favor the idea. A California Field poll conducted in April 1987 indicates that 64 percent of Californians are for voluntary active euthanasia. A Roper poll conducted in March 1988 indicated that even 61 percent of Catholic parishioners favor physician aid-in-dying.

Q: *Under the new law, how will the patient make his or her wishes known?*
A. The patient will sign a DDA directive while competent, witnessed by two disinterested parties, which the patient must make known to the doctor or other health-care provider. The directive is good for seven years, or even longer if the declarant becomes incompetent before the seven-year period ends.

Q: *When will the patient's wish be carried out?*

A: The patient's wish will be carried out when two conditions are fully met. The first is that the patient must be certified as terminal by two licensed physicians, indicating that death is probable within six months. The second condition is that the patient must locate and request a physician who is willing to provide aid-in-dying.

Q: *What happens if the patient becomes comatose or otherwise incompetent?*

A: At the time the DDA directive is signed and witnessed, the patient designates an attorney-in-fact, usually a family member (wife or husband, son, daughter, parent or close friend) to act for him or her in making the health-care decision. This provision is a carry-over of the Durable Power of Attorney for Health Care in the existing law of many States. The attorney-in-fact can then act as a surrogate decision-maker, unless specifically denied this power in the DDA directive. If an attorney-in-fact is not appointed in the directive, the patient's wishes as to life-support systems should be honored by health-care providers.

Q: *Does the law protect physicians and nurses who carry out the patient's wishes?*

A: Yes. The law specifically immunizes and protects physicians and their assistants who follow a patient's direction of all criminal, civil, and administrative liability.

Q: *Isn't the DDA subject to abuse?*

A: As discussed in Chapter Five, it is not subject to abuse any more than any other law. The principal protection against abuse is limiting the number of persons who can provide the assistance to licensed physicians. Doctors are controlled by the state and are professionals guided by standards of ethical conduct. They are trained in the administration of drugs and know better than others how to properly carry out a patient's wish.

Moreover, their economic interests generally run counter to the patient's request. Physicians as well as witnesses must be disinterested, that is, they cannot be heirs, beneficiaries, or creditors of the dying person. Furthermore, decisions by an attorney-in-fact must be reviewed by a three-person ethics committee before the decision can be carried out by the licensed physician. The DDA directive can be revoked at any time by the patient.

Q: *Why have an agent or attorney-in-fact?*

A: The agent may be necessary to carry out a patient's wish if he or she becomes incompetent. However, this is not mandatory or required. Indeed, patients can stipulate that only they, in consultation with their physicians, will decide the time and place of death.

Q: *Isn't it true that medical science may develop a cure for the patient's disease only weeks, days, or even hours after the fatal decision is made?*

A: Medical science has made marvelous advances during the last fifty years, and research and technology continue to move rapidly on all fronts. Yet seldom if ever has a terminally ill patient, as contemplated by the DDA, been saved from death by a last-minute medical discovery. To qualify for the proposed physician aid-in-dying, a patient must be certified as terminally ill by two physicians. Part of their certified judgment must be a consideration of prospective new treatment. Realistically, terminally ill patients who qualify for aid-in-dying under the initiative usually will have had their treatment possibilities exhausted long before the certification. For those who wish to wait until the last breath, hoping for a new medical breakthrough or a divine miracle, aid-in-dying is not for them, and they will not sign directives. The final decision is the patient's. He or she can revoke a directive at the last minute, or the attorney-in-fact (when the patient has become incompetent) can refrain from requesting aid-in-dying for any reason, including the hope that successful new treatment is in sight.

Q: *Isn't this new law the first step toward widespread euthanasia?*
A: Absolutely not. It is a small but reasonable change in the law to permit the dying person relief from his or her final agony and suffering. Moral objections to suicide generally, so-called "mercy killings," or euthanasia in its broadest sense, should not apply to the concept of physician aid-in-dying, as proposed in the initiative. The right to die in a dignified and humane manner, with *the dying individual in control*, makes this concept legally and morally sound. Few laws satisfy the moral criteria of all segments of society. This will be no exception. But the built-in safeguards, particularly the requirement that aid-in-dying be administered only by, or under the supervision of, licensed physicians, and then only to qualified terminally ill persons, obviates any likelihood that it will be a wedge toward unacceptable expansion of euthanasia. Those of us advocating the passage of this law are morally opposed to suicide and mercy killings by family members as well as widespread euthanasia. There is no justification whatever in taking the life of another person. It is morally justified under the DDA only because it is the dying individual's choice to end his or her agony and suffering when he or she elects.

Q: *How can one possibly know that incompetent patients haven't changed their minds?*
A: It is probably not possible to know whether incompetent persons have changed their minds. However, we can assume that since the cognitive process is stopped, there has been no change since the person signed the DDA directive at a time when his or her mental capacities were functioning. It seems safe to infer that the patient's intentions have not changed. Inferences are often drawn in everyday living as well as in the law. The conclusion that an incompetent's in-

tentions remain the same as expressed when competent is reasonable, as was expressed in the *Quinlan* decision, as well as other court cases.

Q: *Doesn't the new law challenge the "sanctity-of-life" concept?*

A: Life is sacred and should and must be protected, cherished, and valued. But a life that is racked with pain and agony is not the kind of life we cherish above all else. Life is sacred until it becomes terminal and the disease, or pathology, becomes irreversible. At that point, deliverance from pain and suffering becomes a goal of many dying individuals, which should be honored. Sanctity of life, in the view of many, is enhanced when dying people are allowed to choose when, where, and how their suffering and lives shall end. Isn't sanctity of life further enhanced when dying people thoughtfully decide where, when, and how to make their last sacraments, or equivalent? Physician aid-in-dying, as proposed here, emphasizes the dignity of human life and provides full opportunity for one to make decisions about death within the framework of one's own spiritual beliefs.

Q: *Won't this new law encourage generalized suicide?*

A: No. As previously pointed out, it is not illegal to commit or attempt suicide now in any state in the country. It is only illegal to assist a suicide. That law will remain intact.

Therefore, it will remain a felony to assist a suicide unless a request is made to a licensed physician through a properly witnessed DDA directive, which can only be carried out when the person has become terminal under the special terms of the initiative. Actually, control over one's destiny at life's end will enhance the quality of life, and of dying.

Q: *Won't the new law discourage physicians from aggressively treating trauma patients to save their lives?*

A: No. Physicians are trained to differentiate among wide varieties of illnesses and their seriousness. They can and do recognize the difference between those suffering from a disease or trauma, such as injury from an automobile accident that can be treated and healed, and those cases of terminal patients whose treatment would only prolong the agony. Physicians will surely not be discouraged from using every heroic measure to save a person who is not terminal and who has not requested assistance-in-dying.

Q: *Isn't it possible that physicians will be mistaken in their prognosis or diagnosis?*

A: Yes. Physicians are fallible human beings just like the rest of us. The Death with Dignity Act anticipates this problem and requires an opinion of a second consulting physician who must concur in the diagnosis and prognosis. It is only then that the patient becomes qualified to request the physician for aid-in-dying. More importantly, the DDA places the responsibility of mistake squarely on the patient, who is required to acknowledge that a physician's judgment is fallible, that it is not always certain but that recognizing these limitations, nevertheless, the patient wishes to proceed with the request for aid-in-dying.

Q: *Will the physician/patient relationship be weakened or compromised if the Death with Dignity Act is enacted?*

A: No. Absolutely not. Complying with a dying patient's request for relief and the physician's ability to comply legally with the request increases the patients' and their families' faith and belief in their physician. The relationship will be strengthened knowing that they are able to relieve the pain and agony of the final dying process, if necessary. After the law is enacted, physicians will not be required to refuse assistance or render it surreptitiously as occurs now. Passage of the act will therefore improve the physician/patient relationship.

Q: *Will physicians who comply with a patient's request under the Death with Dignity Act be violating the Hippocratic oath?*

A: The oath requires a physician to prescribe regimen for

the good of their patients and never do harm to anyone. Complying with a dying person's enduring request for relief from suffering and the indignities of the dying process is not harmful. It is helpful. Moreover, the medical profession has not blindly followed the dictates of the oath over the centuries, but applied common sense and understanding.

Q: *Euthanasia was the first step toward mass genocide in Nazi Germany. Isn't that a possibility in the United States?*

A: It is an extremely remote possibility, as the United States is not Nazi Germany, nor are Americans Nazis. We all know, however, that laws can be abused by government as well as individuals. That is true today without enactment of the Death with Dignity Act. Changing the law to permit and provide an individual autonomous person the right to control his own destiny at life's end does not increase the risk to the rest of us. The Act specifically prevents aid-in-dying to anyone simply because they are a burden to anyone.

Q: *How do doctors stand on the DDA?*

A: Some medical professionals oppose the DDA. Some medical societies like the California Medical Association are also opposed. However, some, like the San Francisco Medical Society, are in favor of the act as it was embodied in the California Initiative Petition. Moreover, there are a large number of doctors in the California Medical Association who support the DDA or reasonable variations thereof. The California Association of Psychologists supports the DDA. There will no doubt be many other associations throughout the country who will support the Act, as time passes.

WIDENER UNIVERSITY-WOLFGRAM LIBRARY

CIR   KF3827.E87 R57 1989
Death with dignity : a new law permittin

3 3182 00306 1337

DISCARD